Captain Ka
– and the –
Malt of Doom

Written in English and Esperanto by Alex Vaughn Miller

This book is dedicated to my parents:

Mi dediĉas ĉi tiun libron al miaj gepatroj:

Randy L. Miller & Wendy L. Miller (Holm)

Text and Illustrations, Copyright © 2017 Alex Vaughn Miller

All rights reserved. / Ĉiuj rajtoj rezervitaj.

ISBN: 1547209526 ISBN-13: 978-1547209521

No part of this publication may be reproduced, stored in a retrieval system, or transmitted, in any form or by any means, electronic, mechanical, photocopying, recording, or otherwise, without the prior permission in writing of the publisher and/or author, or as expressly permitted by law.

Neniu parto de ĉi tiu eldonaĵo povas esti reproduktita, konservita en retrovsistemo, aŭ transmisiita, laŭ ia ajn formo aŭ pere de ia ajn rimedo, elektronika, mekanika, fotokopia, registra, aŭ alia, sen skribita antaŭpermeso de la eldonisto kaj/aŭ aŭtoro, aŭ kiel eksplicite permesata laŭleĝe.

PREFACE IN ENGLISH

I had no idea that malted milk had gluten in it until I learned about celiac while writing Captain Katie's first book. If I was clueless, I figured others might be too so I wrote this story to warn people how dangerous it can be to assume a snack is safe when someone has an allergy. While the villain in this book knows what he's doing, I could see people innocently sharing food with a friend and putting them in danger by accident. This book can help people learn about food safety in a fun (and hopefully preventative) way.

Each of my books includes an Esperanto version of the story along with a translation guide. Esperanto was created in 1887 to be the easiest language on earth to learn. People speak it all over the world and if you learn it, you can stay with Esperantists for free when you travel using a program called Pasporta Servo. Learning it also helps you learn additional languages like Spanish and French more quickly. Check out www.lernu.net/en or visit my YouTube channel *Exploring Esperanto* to learn more. To help support my Esperanto projects and the writing of future books, check out www.Patreon.com/ExploringEsperanto. The last page of this book shows a list of my current patrons.

Alex Vaughn Miller
Lynchburg, Virginia
July 16, 2020

~~~~~~

ANTAŬPAROLO EN ESPERANTO

Mi tute ne sciis, ke malto enhavas glutenon ĝis kiam mi studis celiakion por verki la unuan libron pri Kapitano Katarino. Se mi ne sciis tion, mi supozas, ke tiu informo ankaŭ mankas al aliaj, do mi verkis ĉi tiun rakonton por averti, ke oni ne devus supozi, ke trinkaĵoj aŭ desertoj estas sendanĝeraj, se oni havas alergion.

Kvankam la fiulo en la rakonto komprenas tion, kion li faras, estas komprenebla, ke infanoj povus senkulpe donaci ion glutenan al amikoj hazarde. Per ĉi tiu libro ni povas eduki homojn pri nutraĵa sekuro per amuza (kaj espereble preventa) metodo. Por ekscii kion mi nun faras, abonu mian jutuban kanalon *Esplori Esperanton* aŭ fariĝu patrono ĉe www.Patreon.com/ExploringEsperanto. La fina paĝo de la libro montras liston de miaj nunaj patronoj.

<div align="right">
Alekso MILLER
Linĉburgo, Virginio
La 16an de julio 2020
</div>

Jen aliaj dulingvaj libroj de Alekso MILLER!

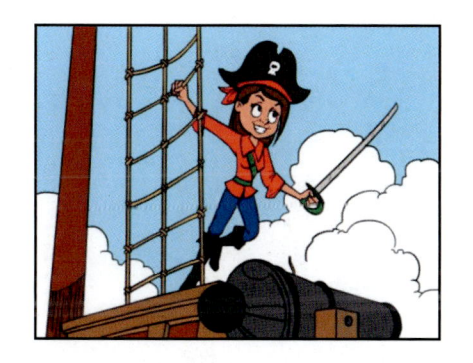

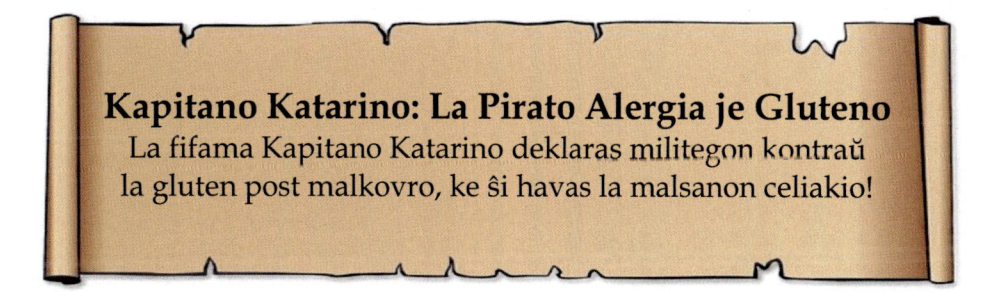

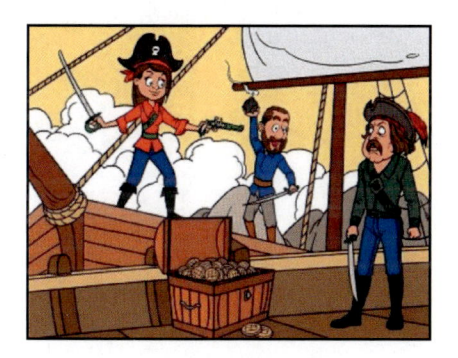

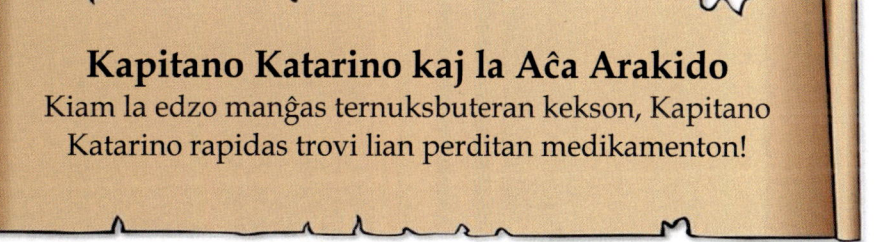

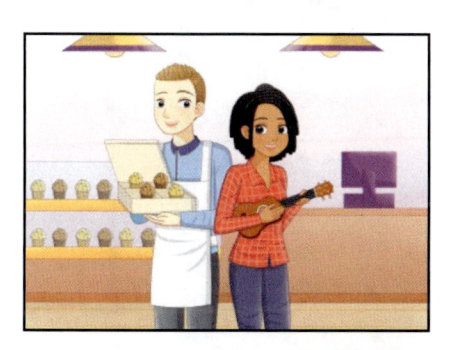

Kapitano Katarino: La Pirato Alergia je Gluteno
La fifama Kapitano Katarino deklaras militegon kontraŭ la gluten post malkovro, ke ŝi havas la malsanon celiakio!

Kapitano Katarino kaj la Aĉa Arakido
Kiam la edzo manĝas ternuksbuteran kekson, Kapitano Katarino rapidas trovi lian perditan medikamenton!

La Nupto de l' Mufenvendisto
Knabo en mufen-kostumo enamiĝas al muzikistino kaj ili kune lernas la gravecon de pensado nekutima!

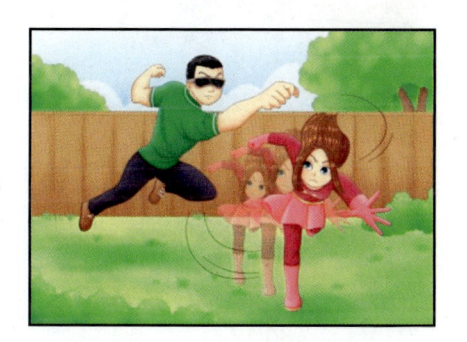

Malplejoto kaj la TroDa Roboto
Kiam potenca nova ordiga roboto agas freneze, nur unu eta heroino povas haltigi lin!

Need Some Help?

There are some big words in this book.
If a word is underlined, check the bottom of that page.
There you'll find out what the word means and how to say it.

The Meter That Matters in Piratous Poems

This whole book is a poem, so before you rehearse,
You should know that it rhymes and is written in verse.
While the meter right here would be called anapest,
We'll be using trochaic for all of the rest.

So the odd-numbered parts will be stressed when you read,
And the sample below ought to help you succeed.
If you think you can handle the meter and feet,
Then iamb pretty sure you are in for a treat.

**ON a PI-rate SHIP of TER-ror
THAT would SCARE your HON-est MEN,
LIVED a PI-rate, CAP-tain KA-tie,
WHO would PLUN-der, NOW and THEN...**

Piratous [PIE-ruh-tuss] = has to do with pirates

Anapest [ann-uh-PEST] = when poetry goes "da-da-DUM, da-da-DUM"

Trochaic [troh-KAY-ick] = when poetry goes "DA-da, DA-da, DA-da"

Succeed [suck-SEED] = "do well" or "do a good job"

Iamb [eye-AM] = a piece of poetry or a word that goes "da-DUM" like *portray* or *respect*

Check out these other bilingual books by Alex Vaughn Miller!

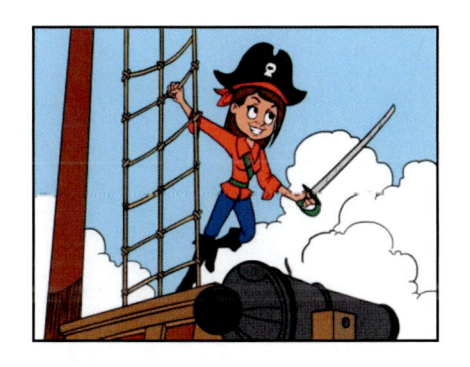

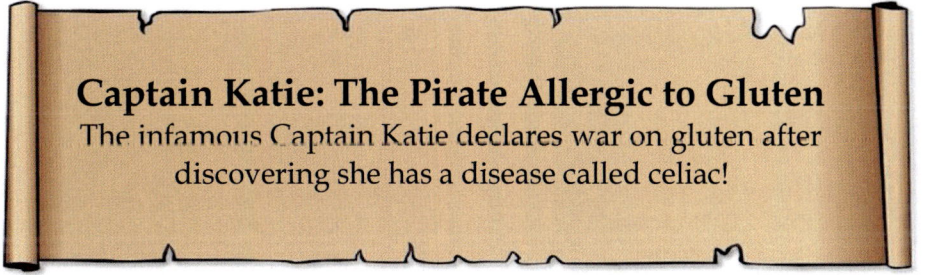

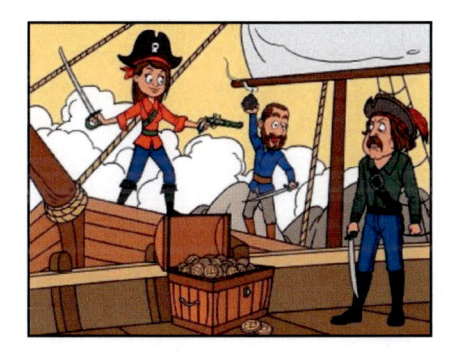

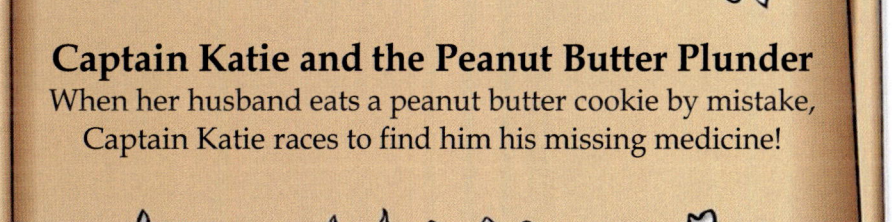

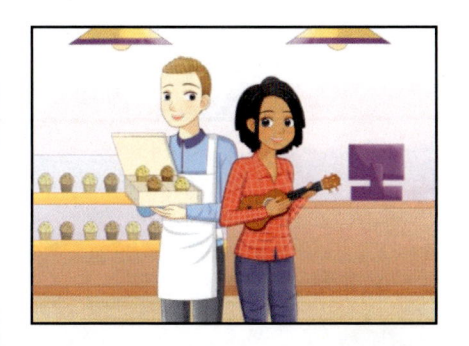

Captain Katie: The Pirate Allergic to Gluten
The infamous Captain Katie declares war on gluten after discovering she has a disease called celiac!

Captain Katie and the Peanut Butter Plunder
When her husband eats a peanut butter cookie by mistake, Captain Katie races to find him his missing medicine!

The Marriage of the Muffin Man
A small town's only ukulele player tries to win a song-writing competition in a faraway city!

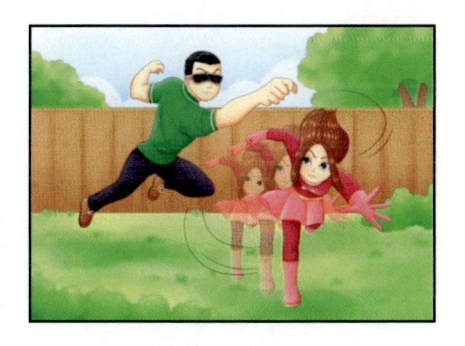

Minnie Miser and the XS Machine
When a powerful new cleaning robot gets out of control, only the mighty Minnie Miser can shut him down!

Captain Katie
and the Malt of Doom

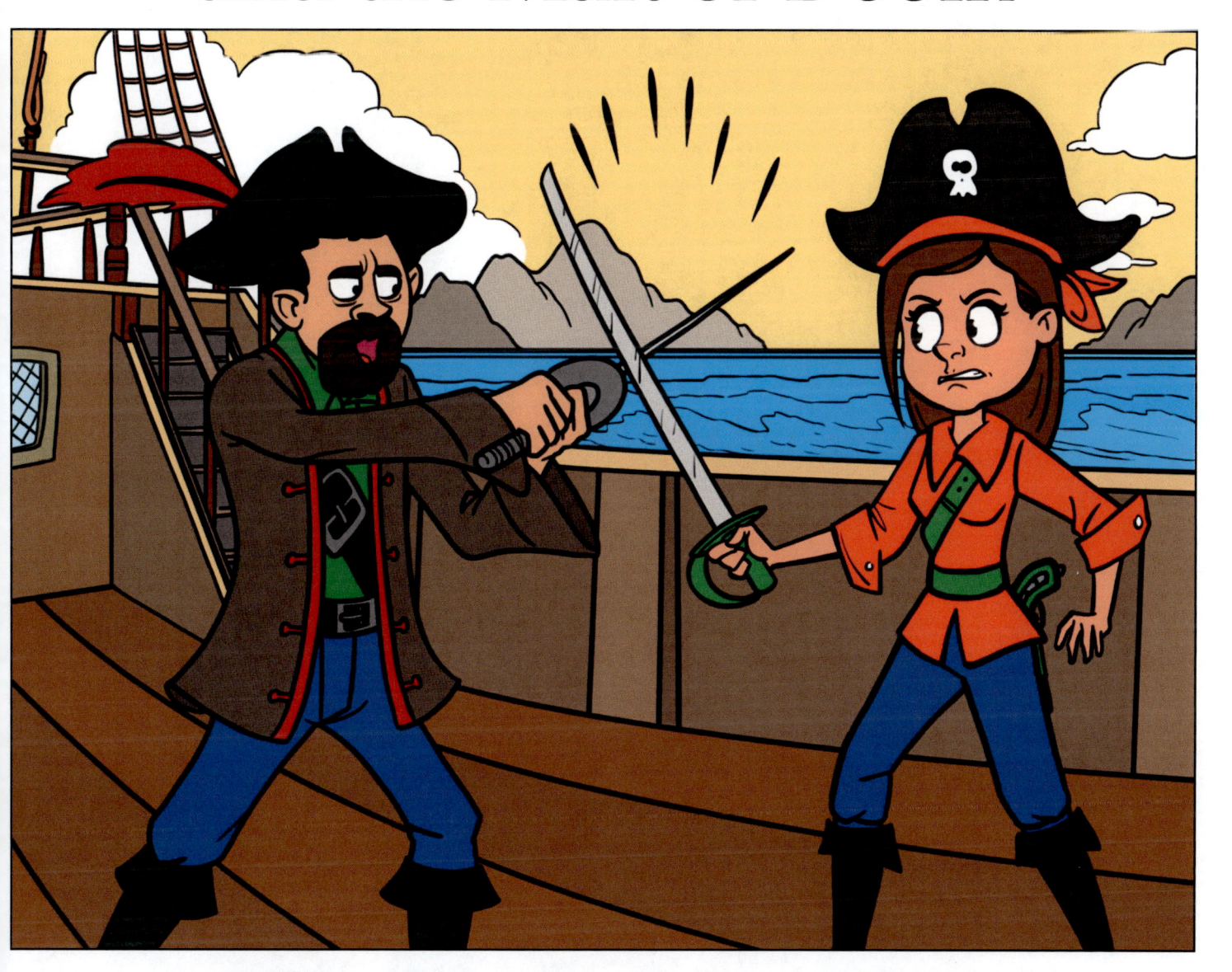

The English Version

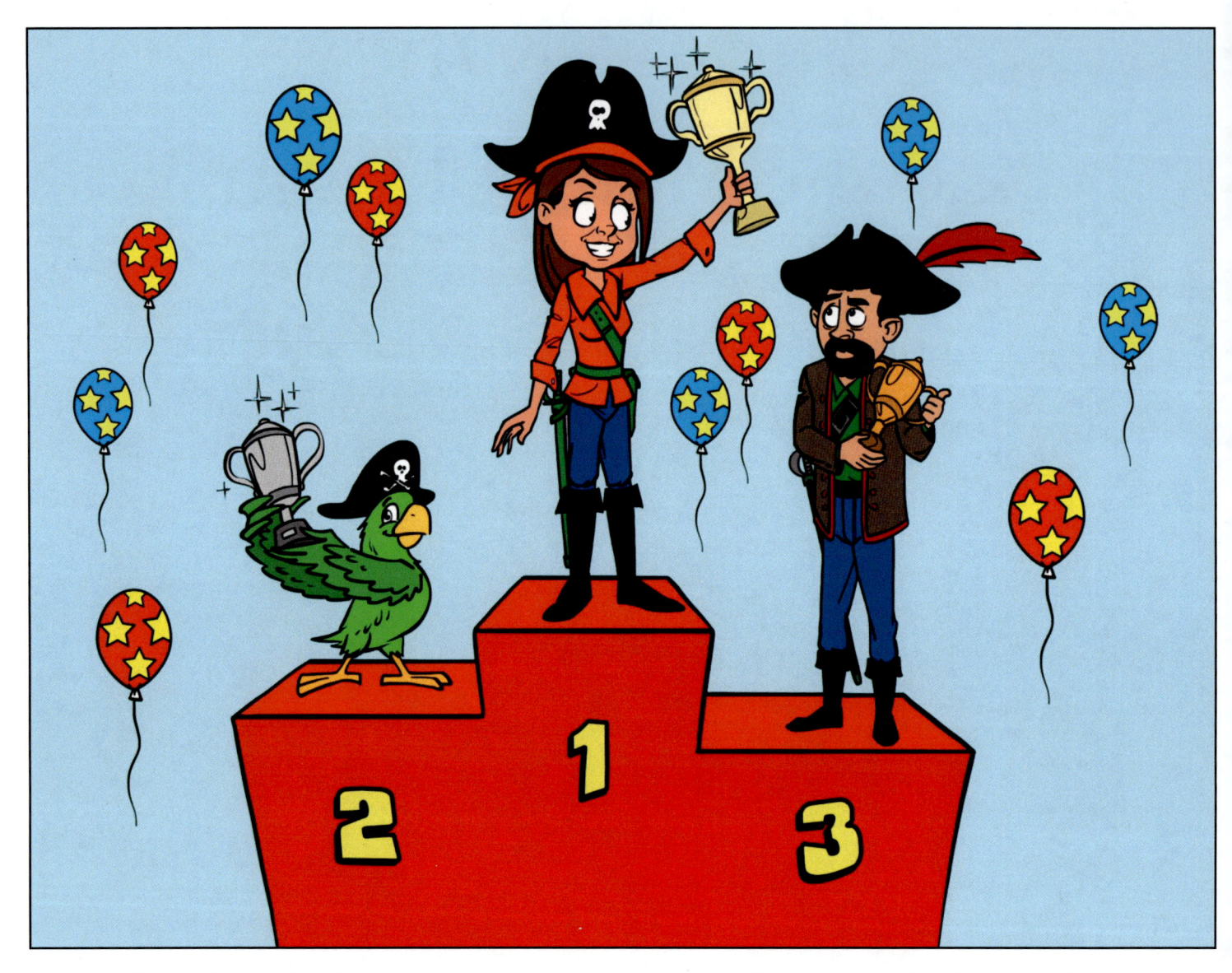

'Twas the day for pirate racing
And the crews were cruising fast,
But the checkered flag finale
Featured Katie unsurpassed.

Poor Commander Robert Barley
Was disheveled and disgraced.
Captain Katie'd won the gold,
Yet Barley's ship had barely placed.

Finale [fin-AL-ee] = the finish, the end of the race

Disheveled [dish-SHEV-vuld] = untidy, in a mess

Placed [PLAYST] = finished the race in first, second, or third place

Unsurpassed [UN-sir-PAST] = unbeaten

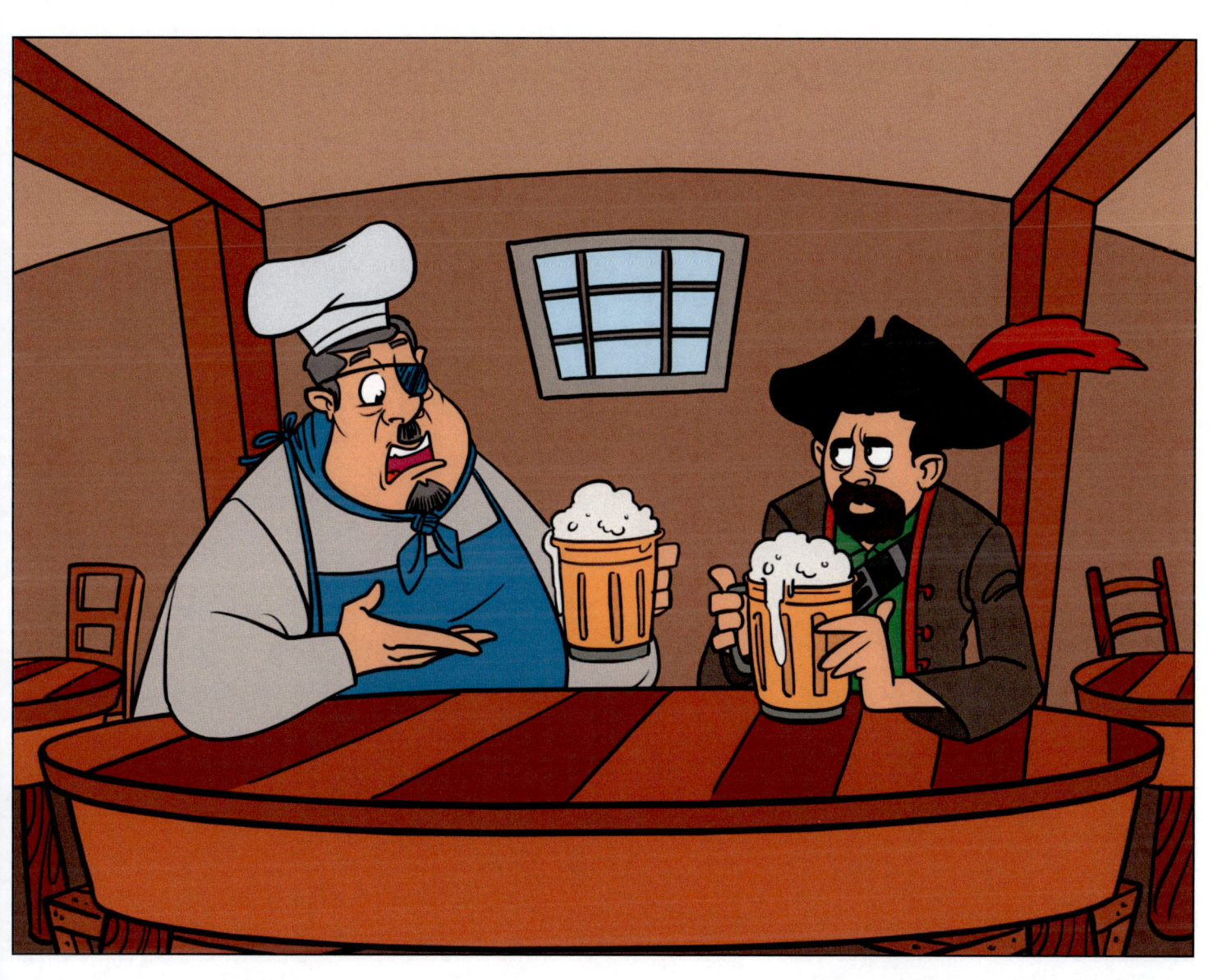

He <u>determined</u> to destroy her
By whatever means he could.
If she only had a weakness,
He'd be rid of her for good!

While he drank his drink at Arrbucks,
Barley heard the chef explain
That if Katie's food had <u>gluten</u>,
She would topple down in pain.

"What is gluten?" Barley asked him,
"I have never seen the word."
"It's a <u>compound</u> some can't handle,
Found in wheat. In fact, I've heard…"

Determined [dee-TUR-minned] = strongly decided

Gluten [GLOO-tin] = a part of some grains like wheat that makes the dough all stretchy

Compound [CAHM-pownd] = a thing made up of two or more things chemically bonded together

3

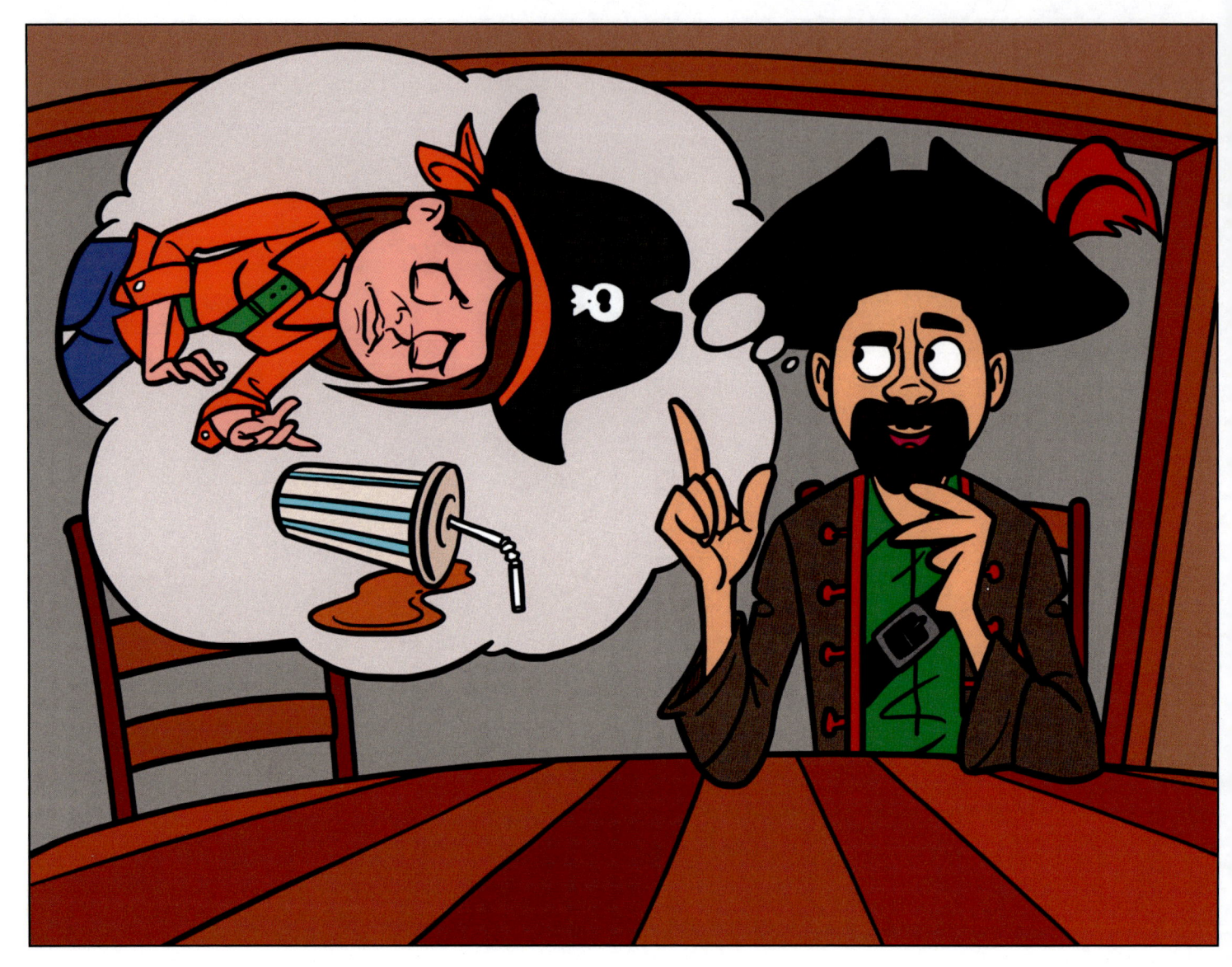

"Certain grains, like triticale,
Several oats, farina, rye,
And the malt that comes from barley,
They could cause the girl to die!"

"Fascinating!" pondered Barley.
He had malted milk galore
That he used when making milkshakes
In his malted milkshake store.

And if Katie didn't question
What he put in what she ate,
With a frozen malt confection,
He could poison Captain Kate!

Triticale [trit-ih-KAY-lee] = a hybrid grain made from wheat and rye
Farina [fuh-REE-nah] = a wheat often used in hot cereal
Confection [kun-FEK-shun] = a treat made with sweet ingredients

Galore [guh-LORE] = aplenty, lots of it

4

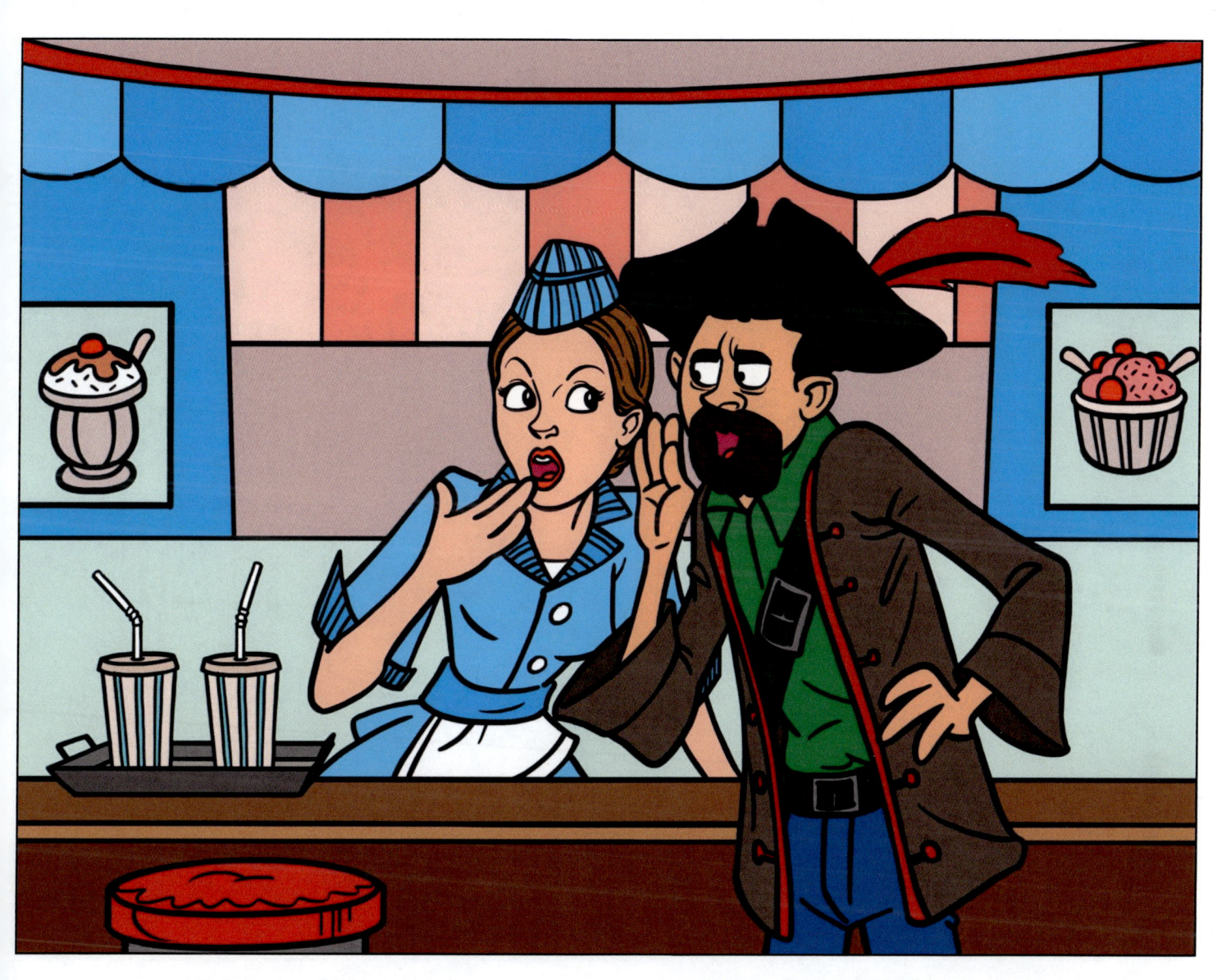

He instructed his assistant
To prepare the deadly treat,
Then appeared a short time later
On a <u>vessel</u> <u>void</u> of wheat.

Knock, knock, knock! "Oh, hello, Katie!"
"There's your husband. Hello, Drew!"
He presented two large milkshakes,
Then he <u>toasted</u>, "Here's to you!"

Vessel [VESS-uhl] = a boat

Void [VOYD] = empty, completely without

Toasted [TOE-stid] = said something nice before sharing a drink

5

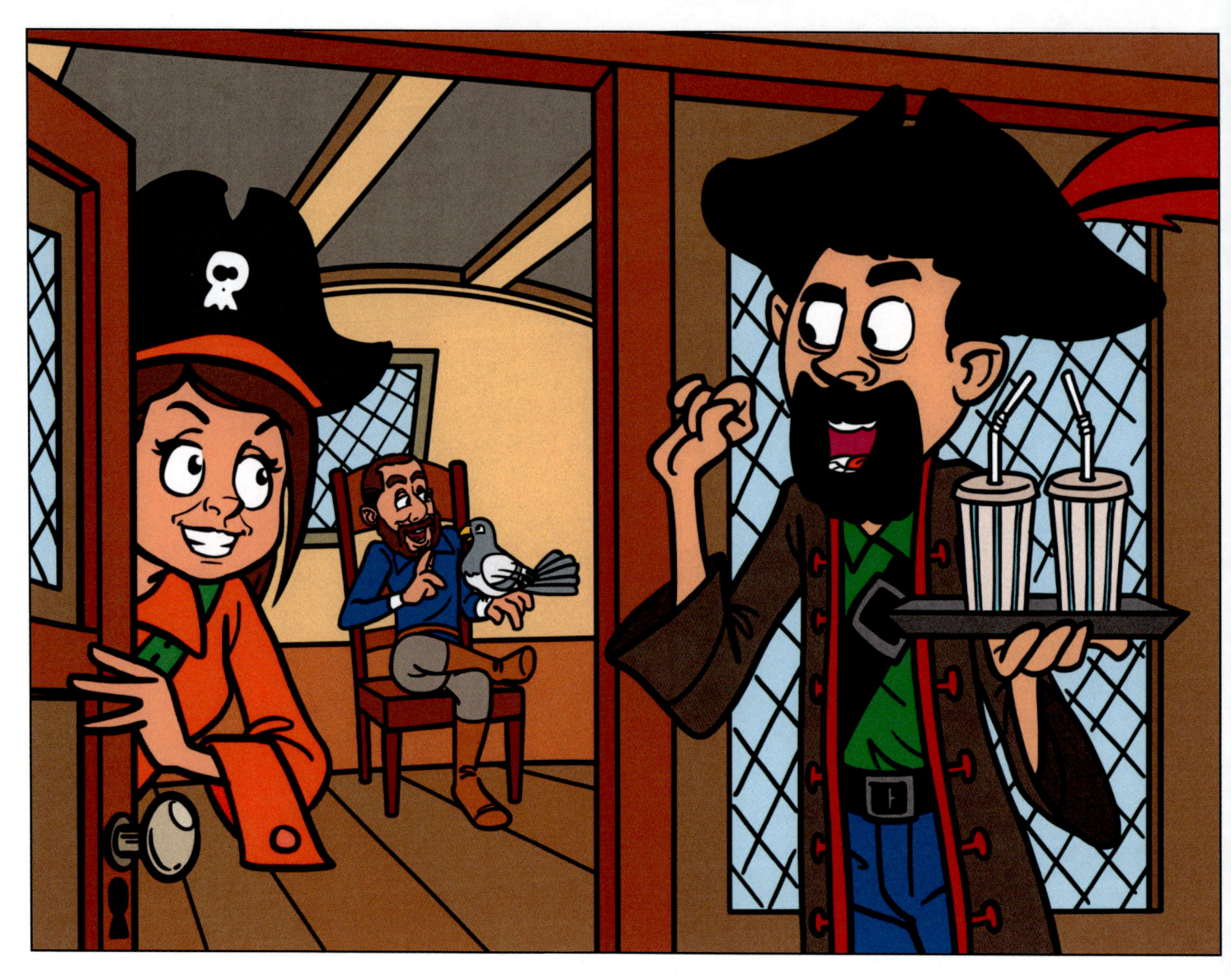

"These are perfect!" answered Katie,
"And there's something ye should know:
We are having our first baby,
So our racing has to go!"

"We both hope you'll win it next year,
And we'll cheer yer team along!
Yer boat's bound to beat the others,
But now— wait. Is something wrong?"

Ye [YEE] = an old-fashioned, pirate way of saying *you*

Bound [BOWND] = definitely will, is sure to

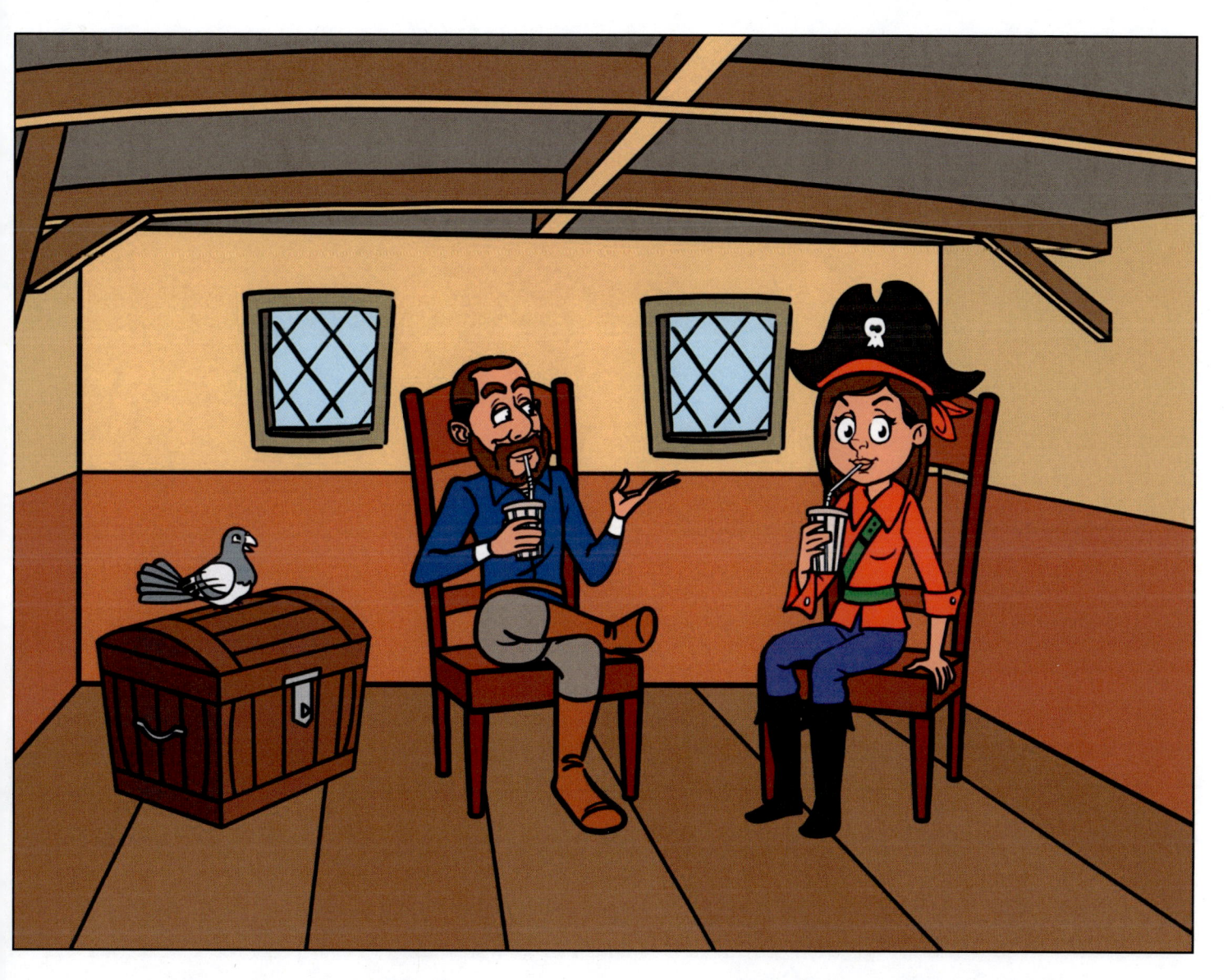

He was glancing at the milkshakes
And deciding what to say,
Yet his pain from losing lingered,
So he simply muttered, "Nay!"

Katie drank her malted milkshake
Just as Barley'd hoped she would,
Then she grasped her belly, belting,
"I don't think I feel so good!"

Lingered [LING-gurd] = had not left, was still there

Belting [BELL-ting] = saying very loudly

7

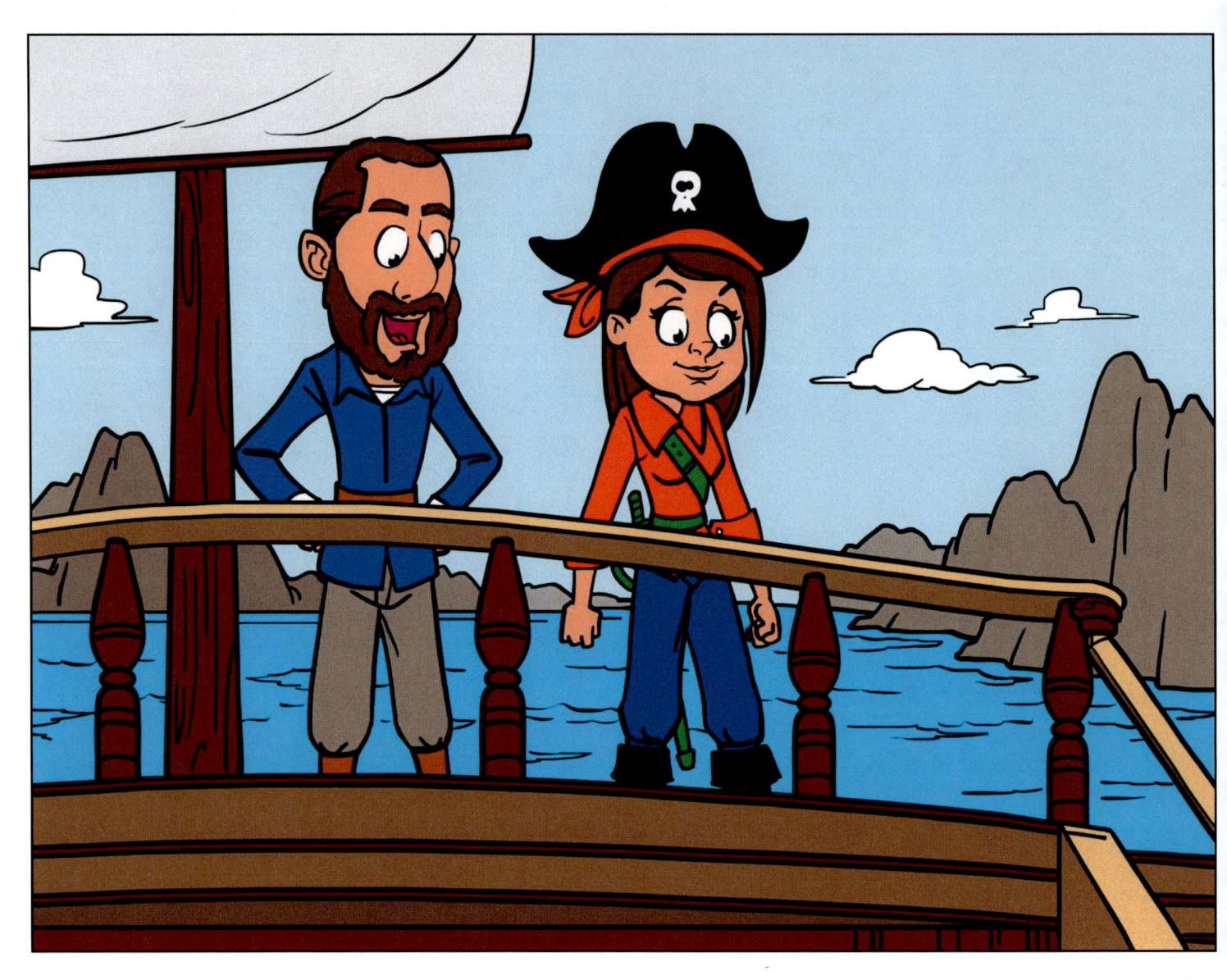

To the quarterdeck they hurried,
To give Katie some fresh air.
Robert Barley stood there smirking
At the couple in despair.

Katie turned to Robert Barley,
Then she stood up, good as new.
"When I told ye I was sick," she said,
"'Twas from the sight of you!"

Quarterdeck [KWOR-ter-dek] = the raised part of the ship where the captain gives the orders

Smirking [SMUR-king] = an irritating, annoying, smug way of smiling

Despair [dih-SPARE] = hopelessness, unhappiness

8

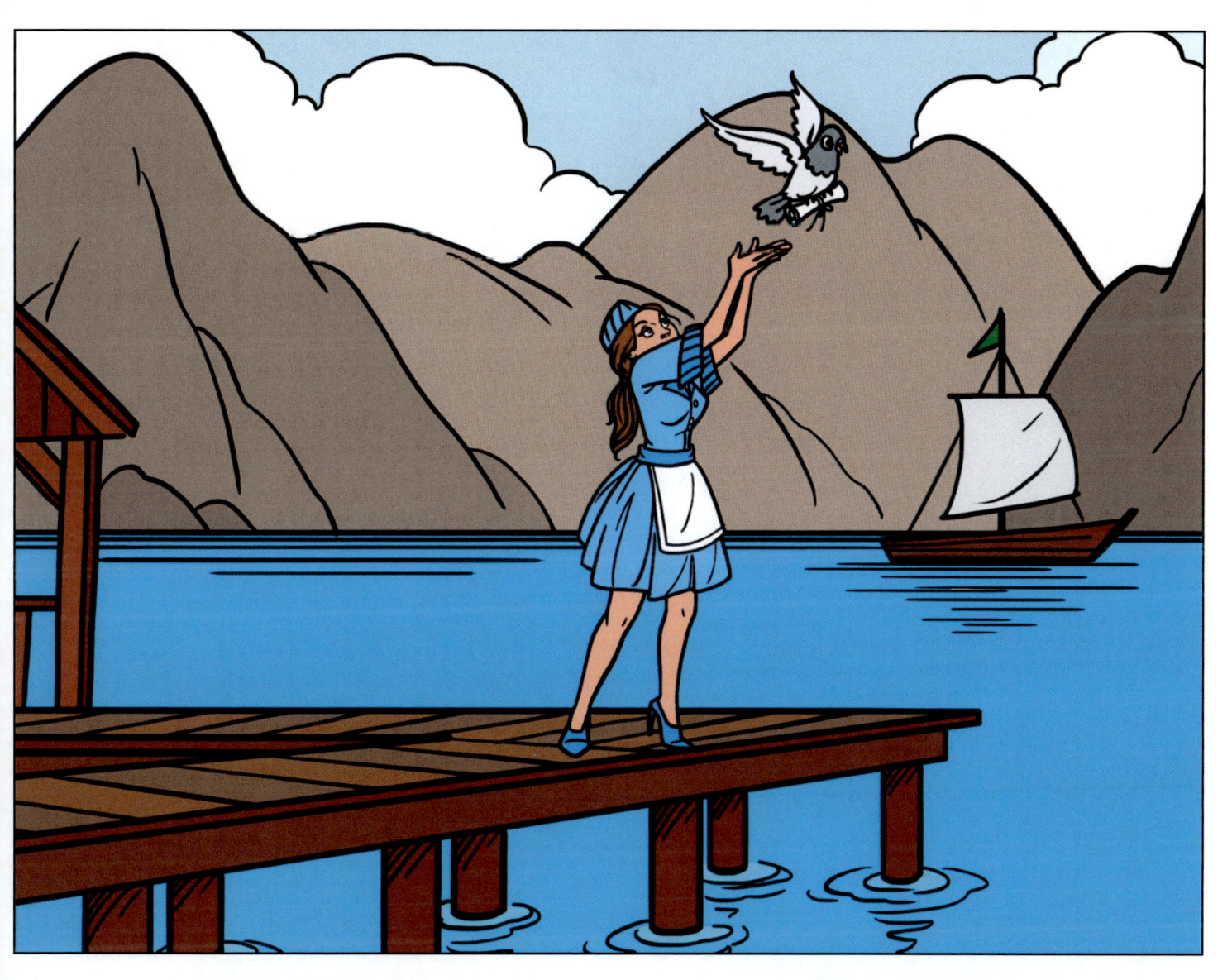

"Yer assistant, Mia Millet,
Sent a pigeon with a note;
Said she swapped me malted milkshake
With a frothy root beer float!"

Robert Barley stared in horror
She had learned his wicked plan!
Then he swore, "I'll still destroy you
With my sword instead of bran!"

Millet [MILL-it] = a grain that does not have gluten in it

Frothy [FRAWTH-ee] = foamy or bubbly

Bran [rhymes with *ran*] = the outer part of a grain (which often has gluten in it)

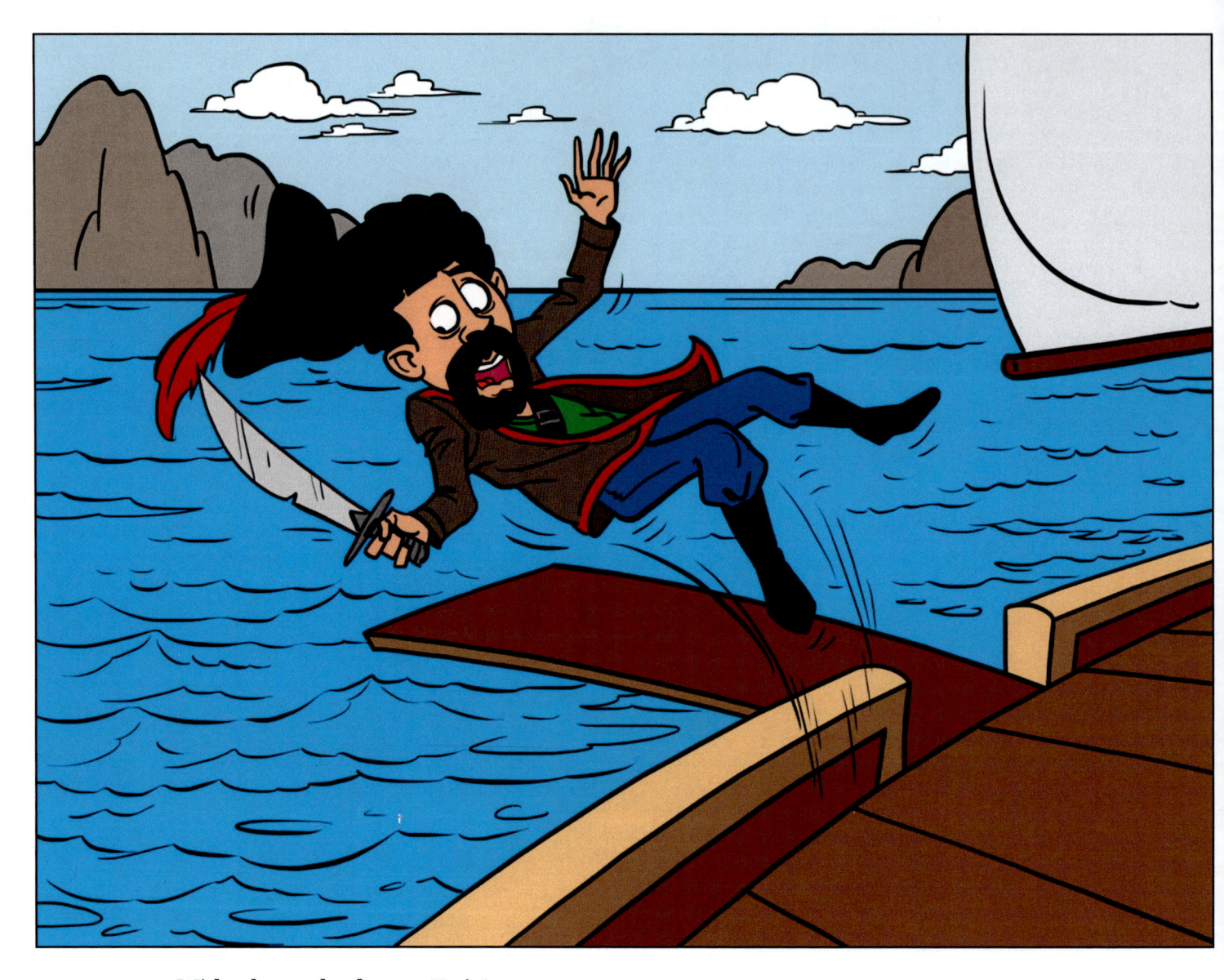

With a <u>lunge</u>, he dove at Katie!
With a step, she dodged the blow!
Drew <u>disarmed</u> him with his dagger.
Toward the plank he pushed his foe.

"I'm a winner!" shouted Robert,
While the waves below him roared.
In his rage, he lost his footing;
Barley tumbled overboard.

Lunge [LUHNJ] = a quick forward move in sword fighting, usually to attack suddenly

Disarmed [diss-ARMD] = took away or made him drop his weapon

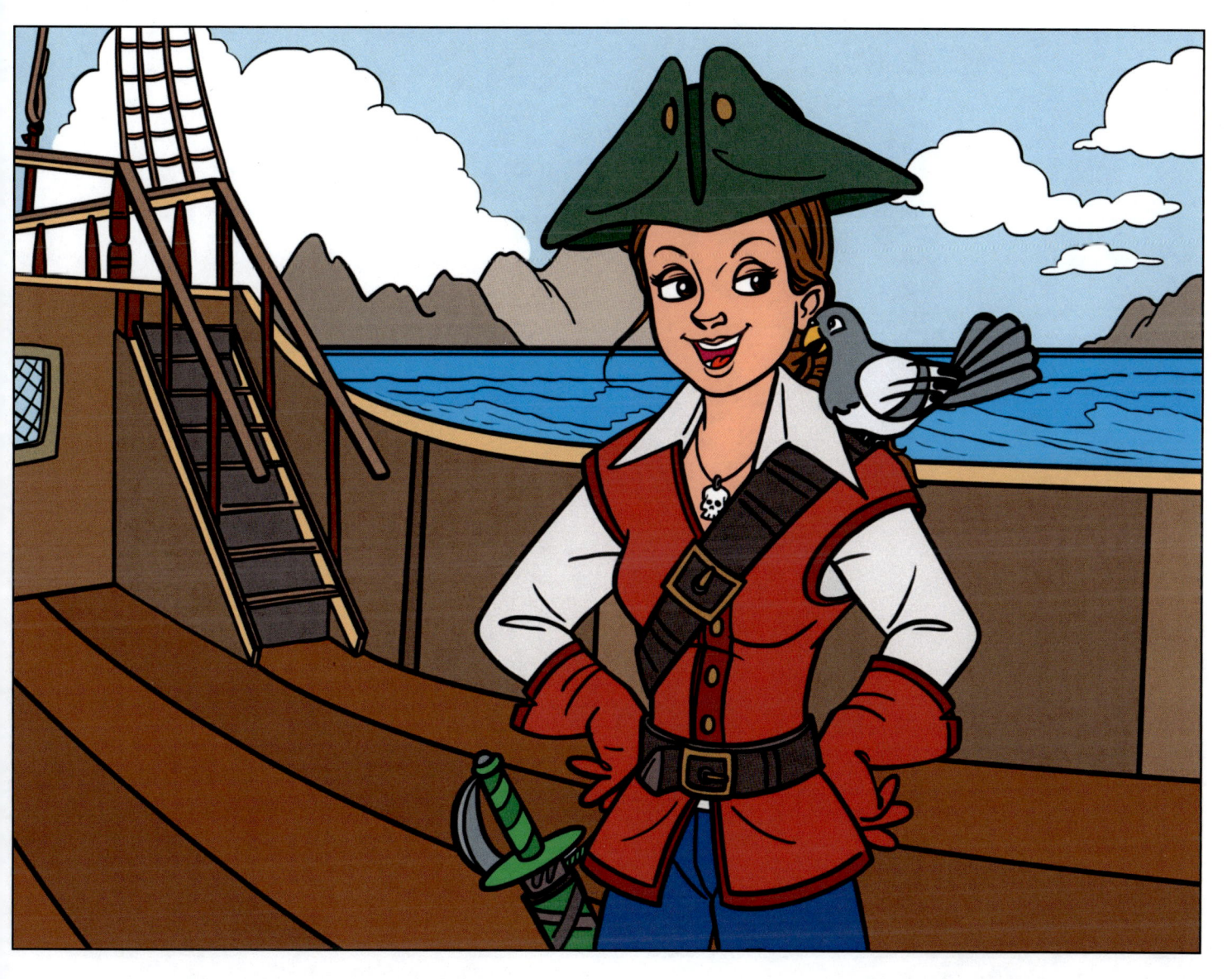

Though they never found his body,
We believe old Robert's dead.
One year later, Captain Mia
Won that <u>golden cup</u> instead.

Barley's boot was given to her
By his crew for being brave,
And she proved, to be a winner,
You don't have to misbehave.

Golden cup = the first-place trophy or prize for winning the pirate race

11

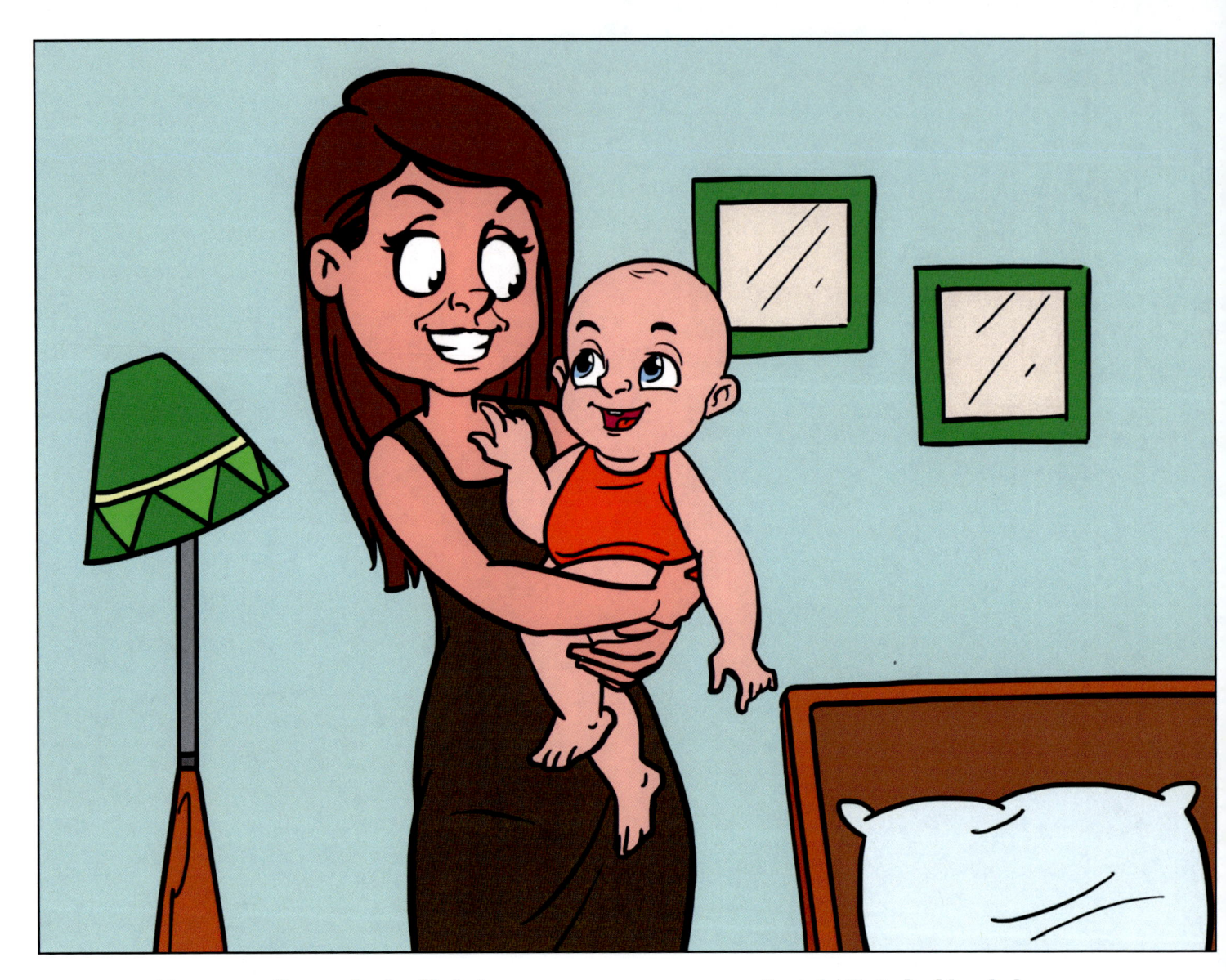

Now, regarding malted milkshakes,
Don't forget to stay alert,
Just in case your friends and family
Can't digest the same dessert.

Captain Katie had her baby
And they lived a lovely life.
Though her claim to fame was pirate,
She excelled as mom and wife.

Regarding [ree-GAR-ding] = "When it comes to…"

Digest [die-JEST] = fully eat

Excelled [ek-SELLD] = did a great job

Want to read that story again in another language?
Just turn the page to get started.
There's a guide in the back of the book to help you do it.

Kapitano Katarino kaj la Malto de Veneno

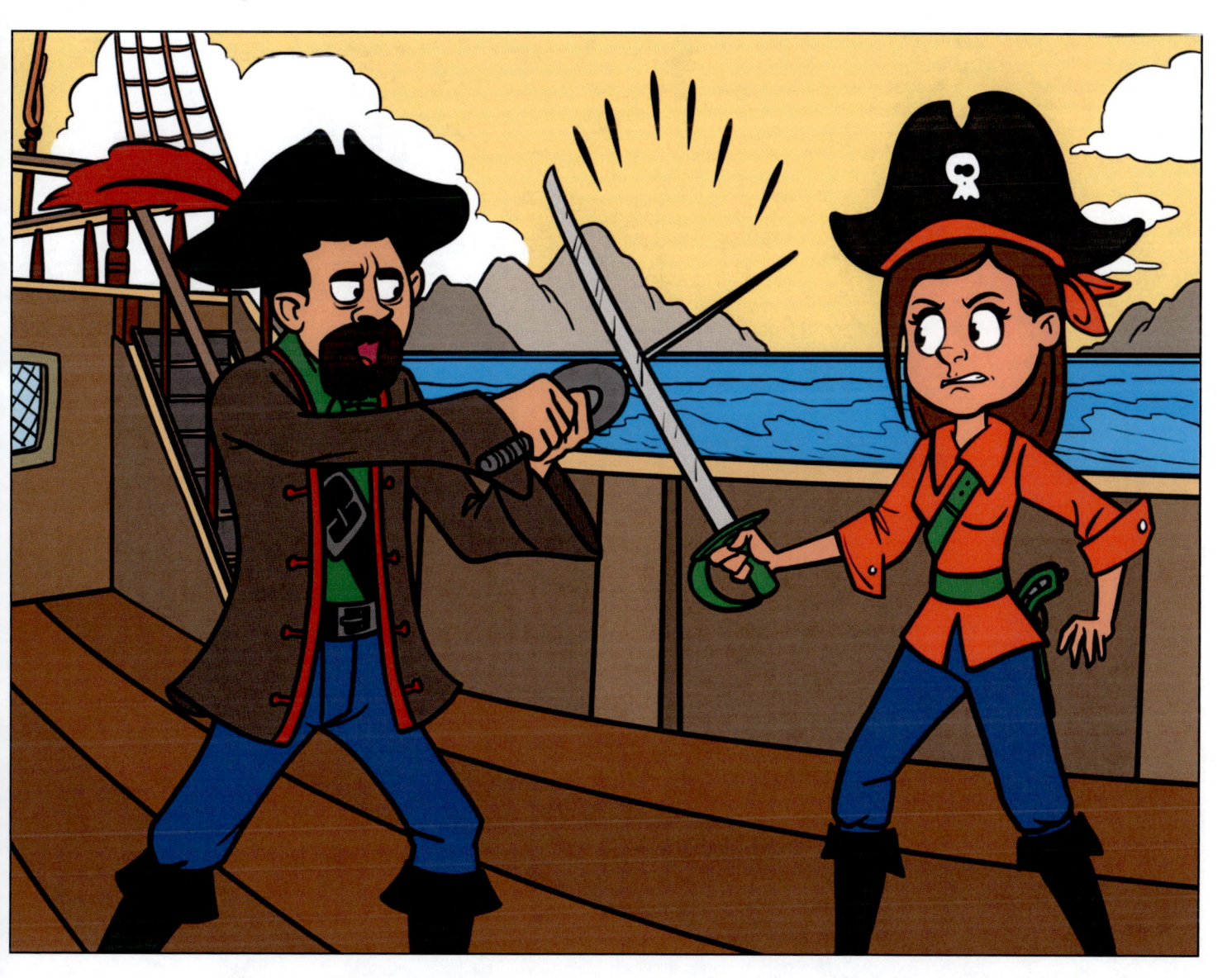

La Esperanto-Versio

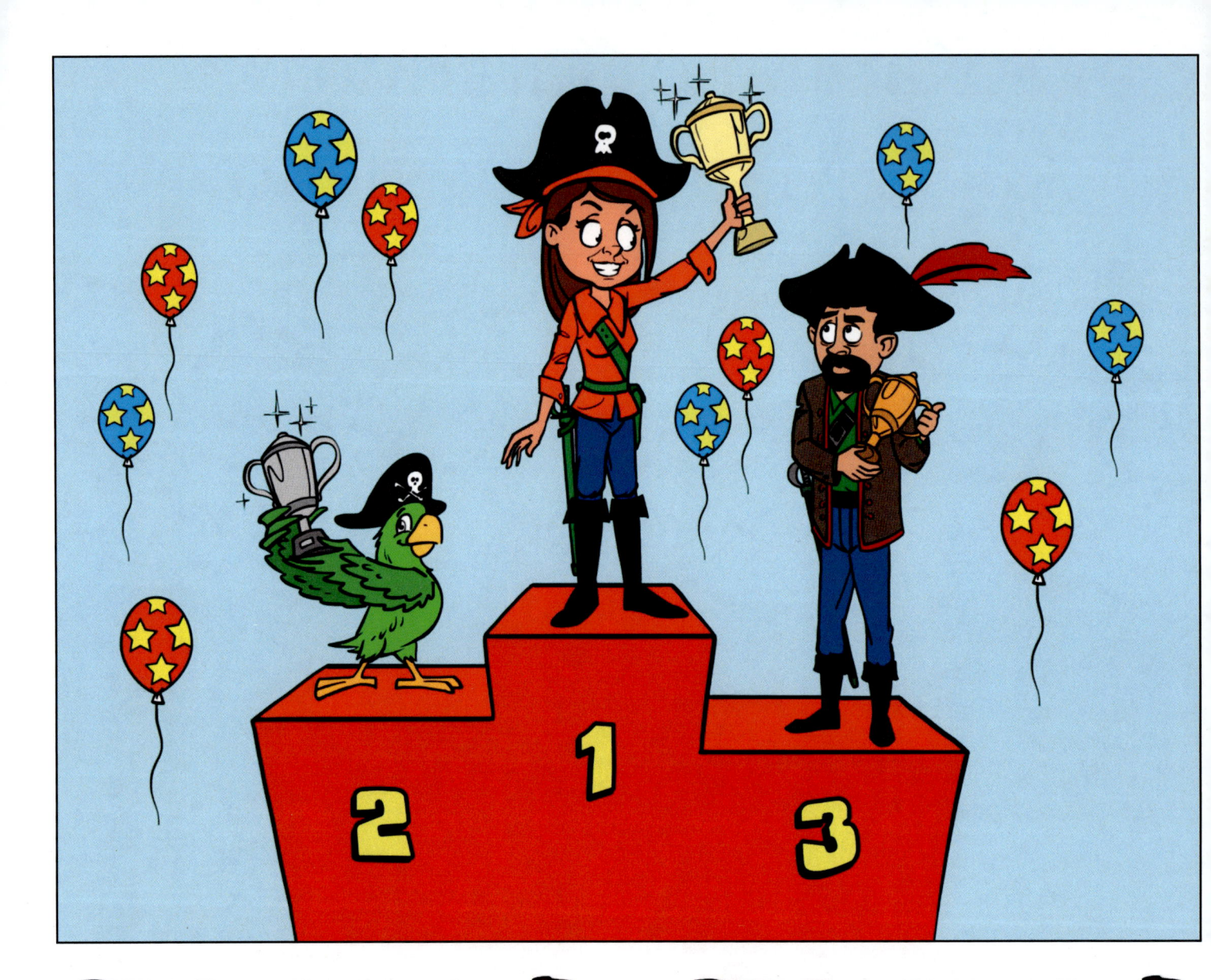

Estis tago por pirata
Ŝipkonkurso, kaj la fin'
Montris, ke la gajnon tenis
Kapitano Katarin'.

Kompatinda Berto hontis
Pro malgajno kontraŭ ŝi.
Ne premion de la oro,
Sed de bronzo gajnis li.

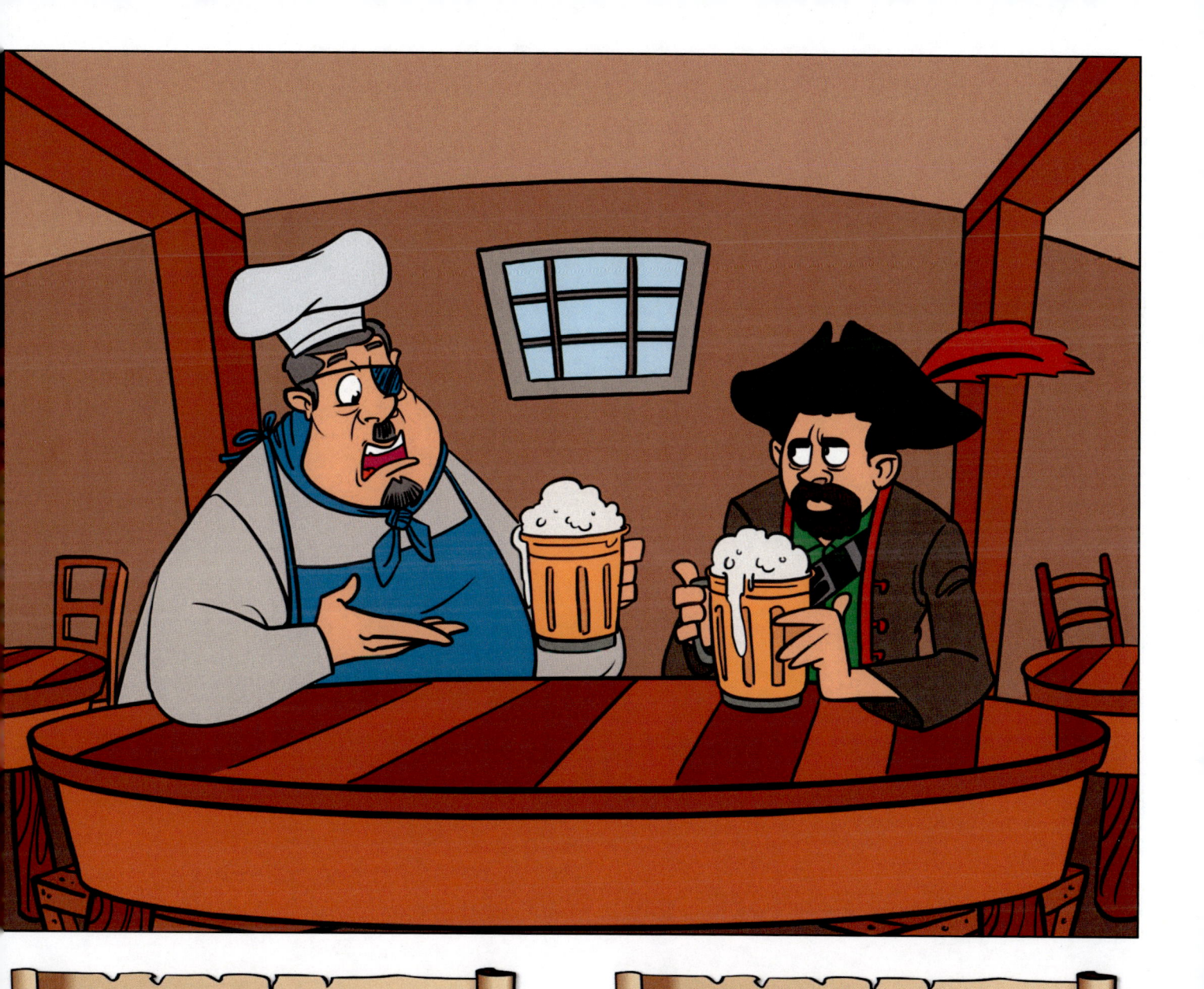

Li decidis ŝin detrui,
Kiel ajn li eble povus.
Se ŝi havus vundeblecon,
Tion certe li eltrovus.

Dum drinkado, Berto aŭdis
Kuiriston, kiu diris,
Ke nur senglutenaj manĝoj
Al Katanjo ĉiam iris.

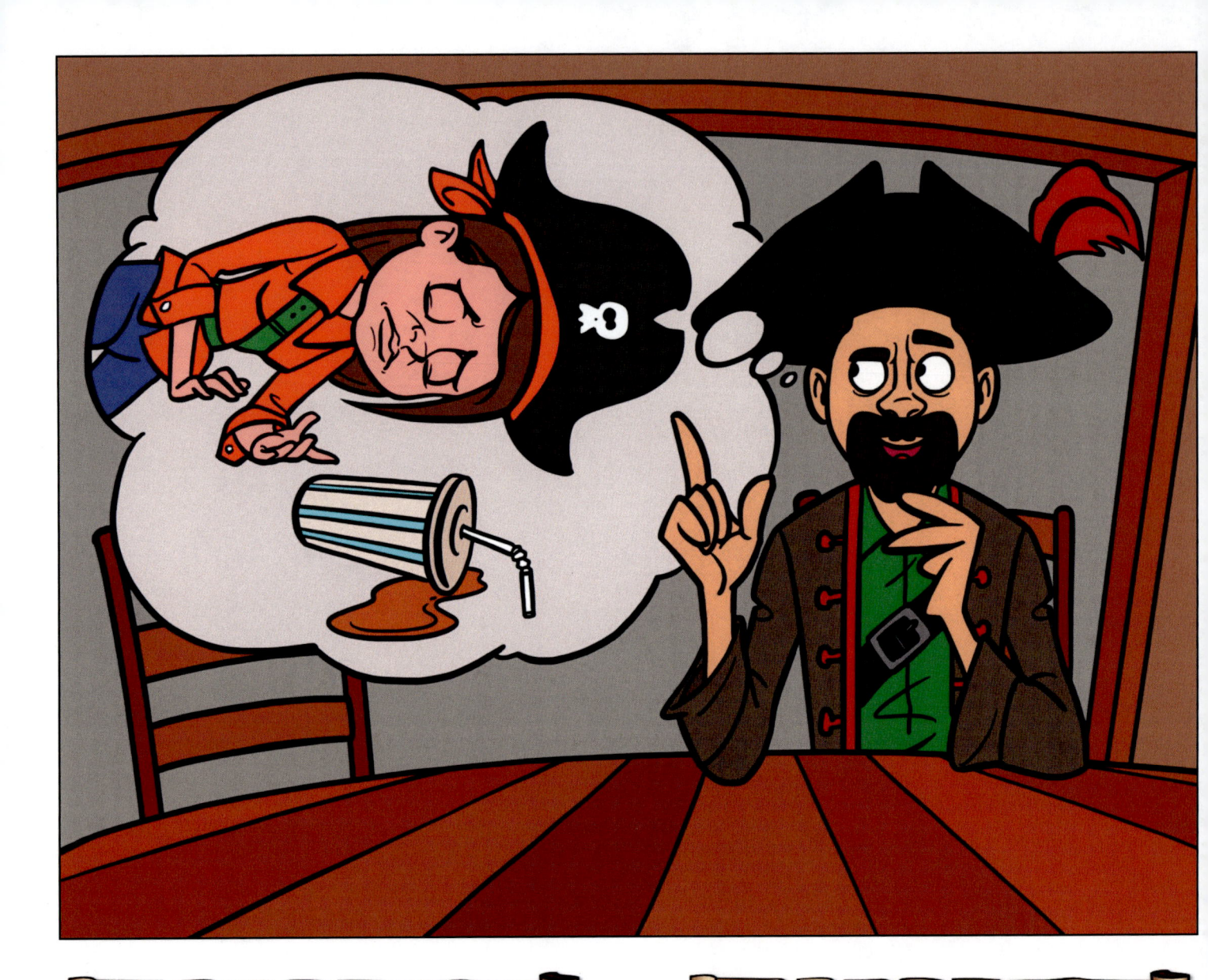

"Ĉu gluteno?" li demandis,
"Mi ne konas la terminon."
"Jen faruna aĵo, kiu
Doloregus Katarinon."

"Ĝi troviĝas en tritiko,
La durumo, kaj sekalo.
Eĉ la malto de hordeo
Sendus ŝin al hospitalo."

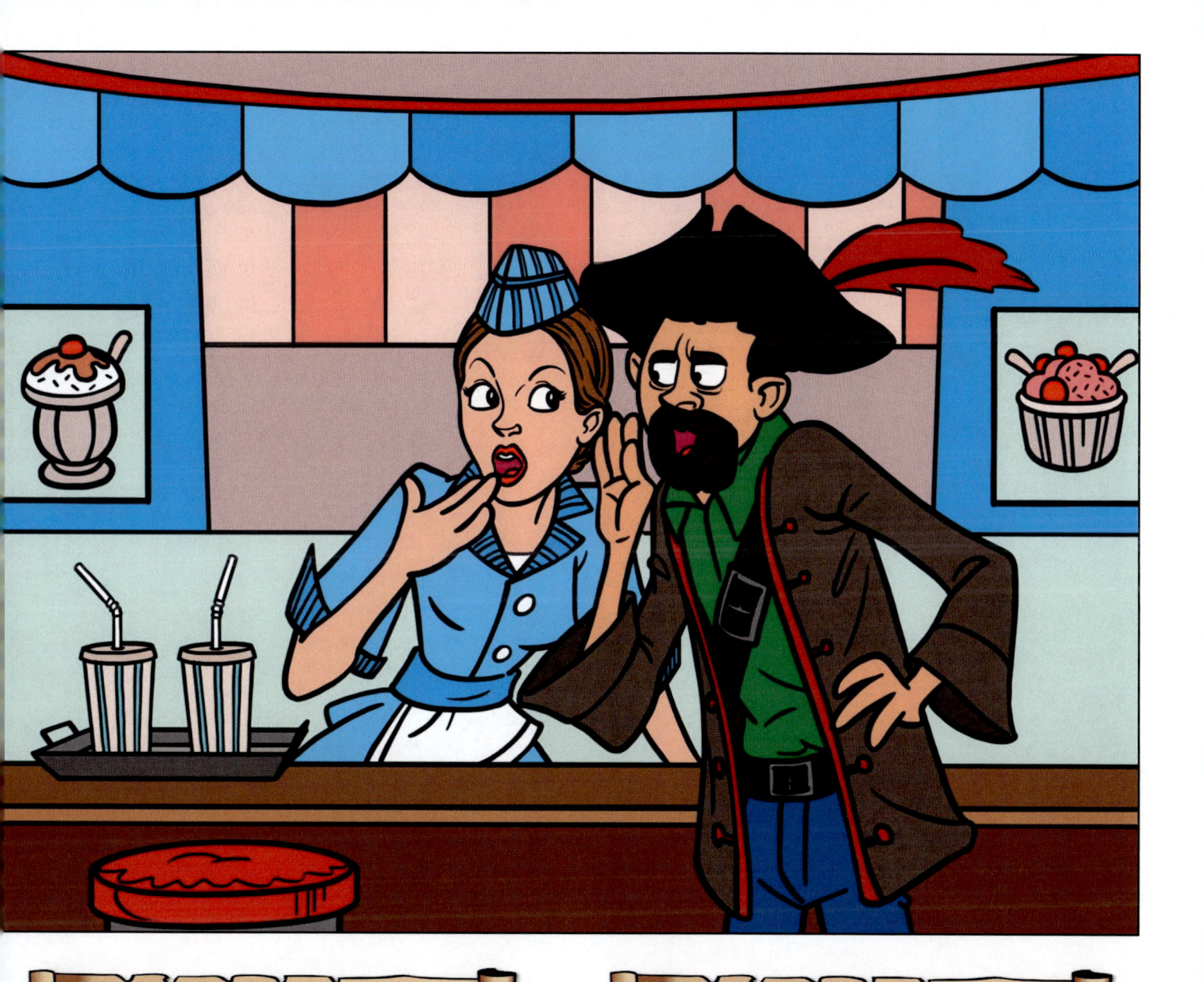

"Interese," pensis Berto,
"Tiun malton, estas fakto,
Oni uzas por kunmiksi
Glaciaĵon kun la lakto."

Se Katanjo ne komprenus,
Ke enhavas malt' glutenon,
Per kirlaĵo, li ŝin donus
Tre venenan glasoplenon.

v

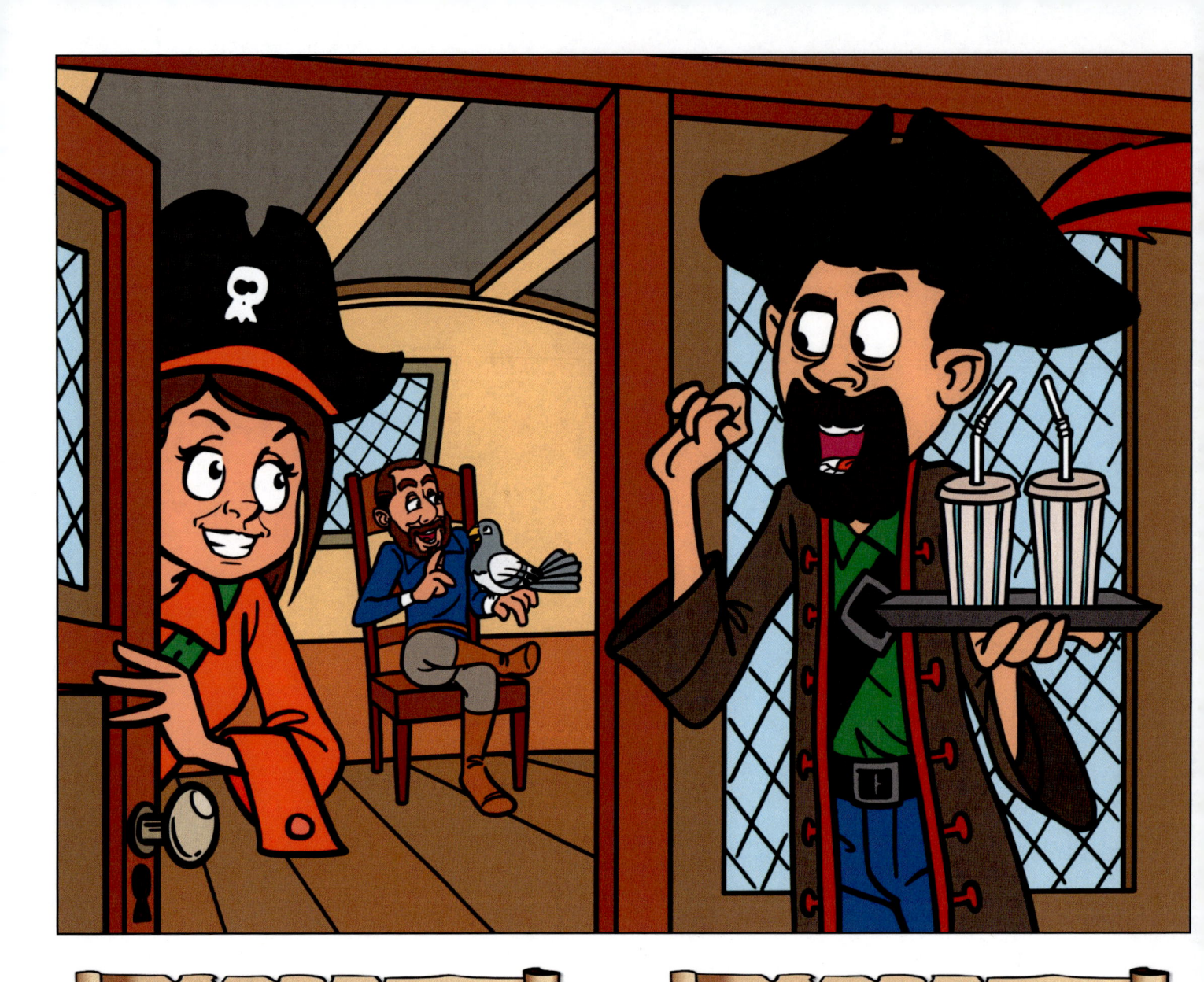

Li de l' kelnerino mendis
Du maltaĵojn de deserto.
Poste al la piratŝipo
De Katanjo iris Berto.

Al Katanjo kaj al Druo,
Ŝia edzo, donis li
La trinkaĵojn, kun la tosto,
"Je la venko kontraŭ mi!"

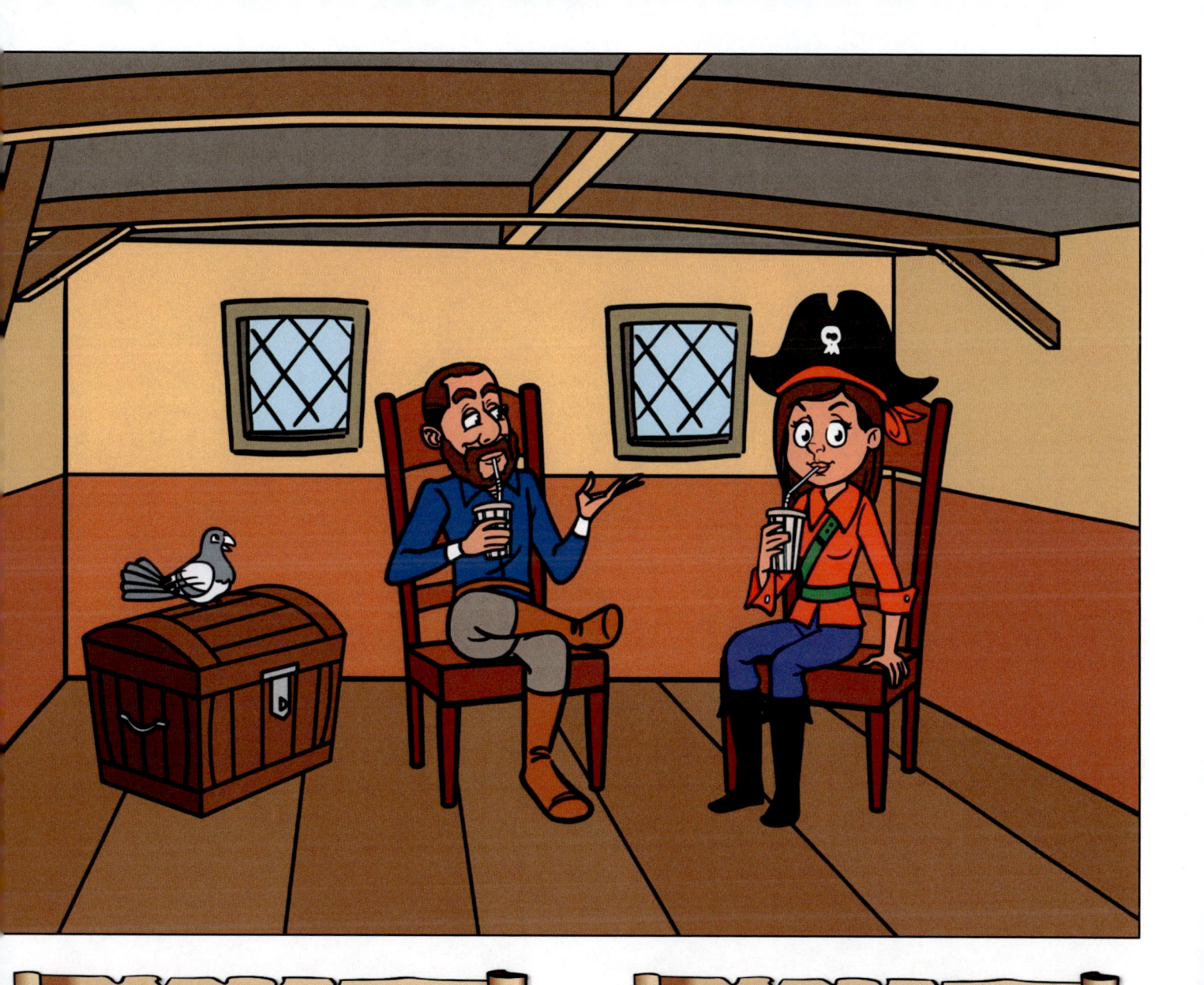

"Dankon, Berto! Kaj aŭskultu!
Mi graveda estas. Vere!
Konkursado mia ĉesos,"
Diris ŝi al li sincere.

Ĉu li devus ŝin informi
Pri la malto de horde'?
La malgajn' lin kolerigis
Do li simple pensis, "Ne."

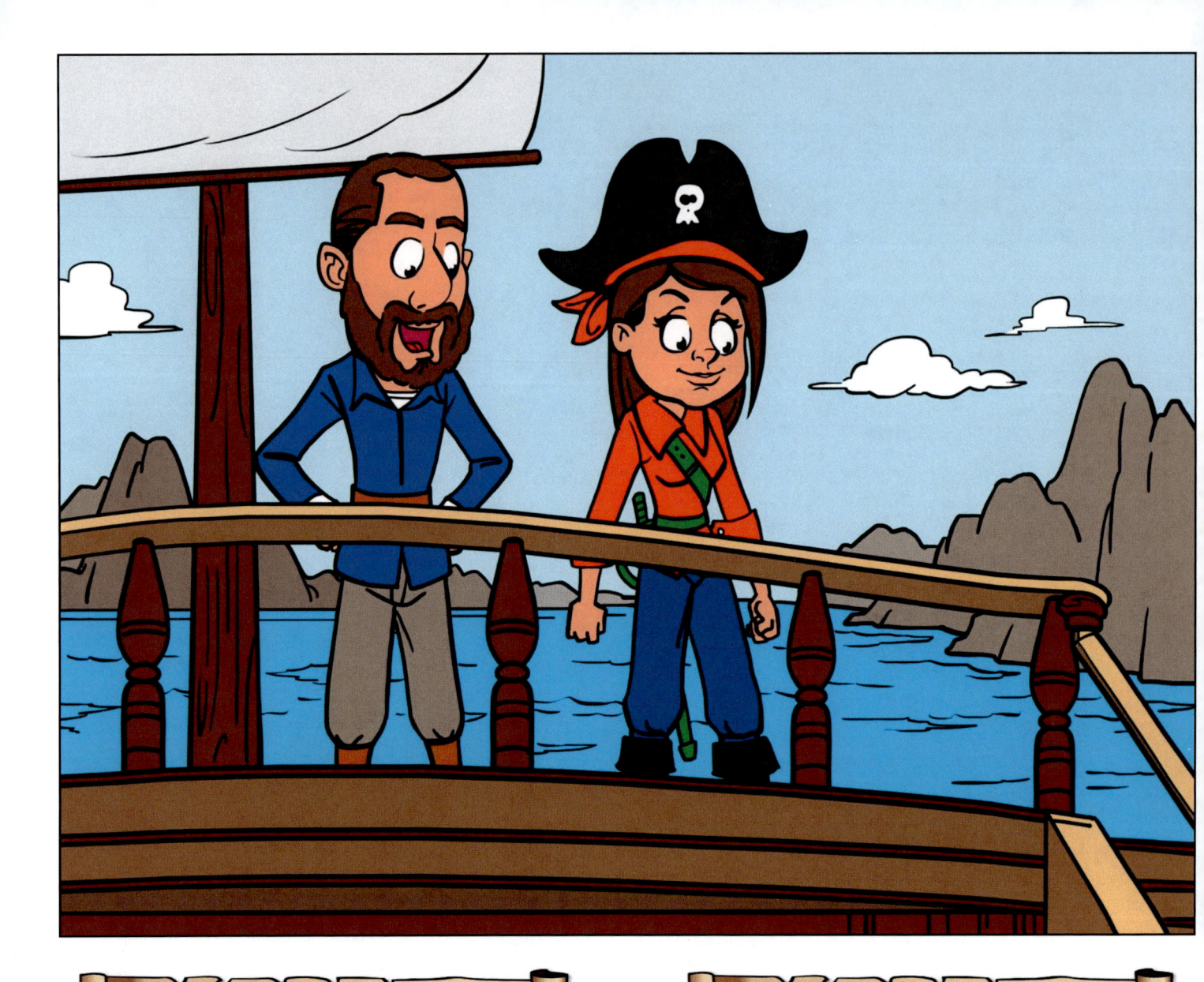

Ŝi fortrinkis la deserton.
Kaj sin tenis per la mano.
Berto ridis dum ŝi diris,
"Kien iris mia sano?"

"Mi eksteren devas iri!"
Do la viroj sekvis ŝin.
Berto ĝojis en la koro
Pro l' dolor' de Katarin'.

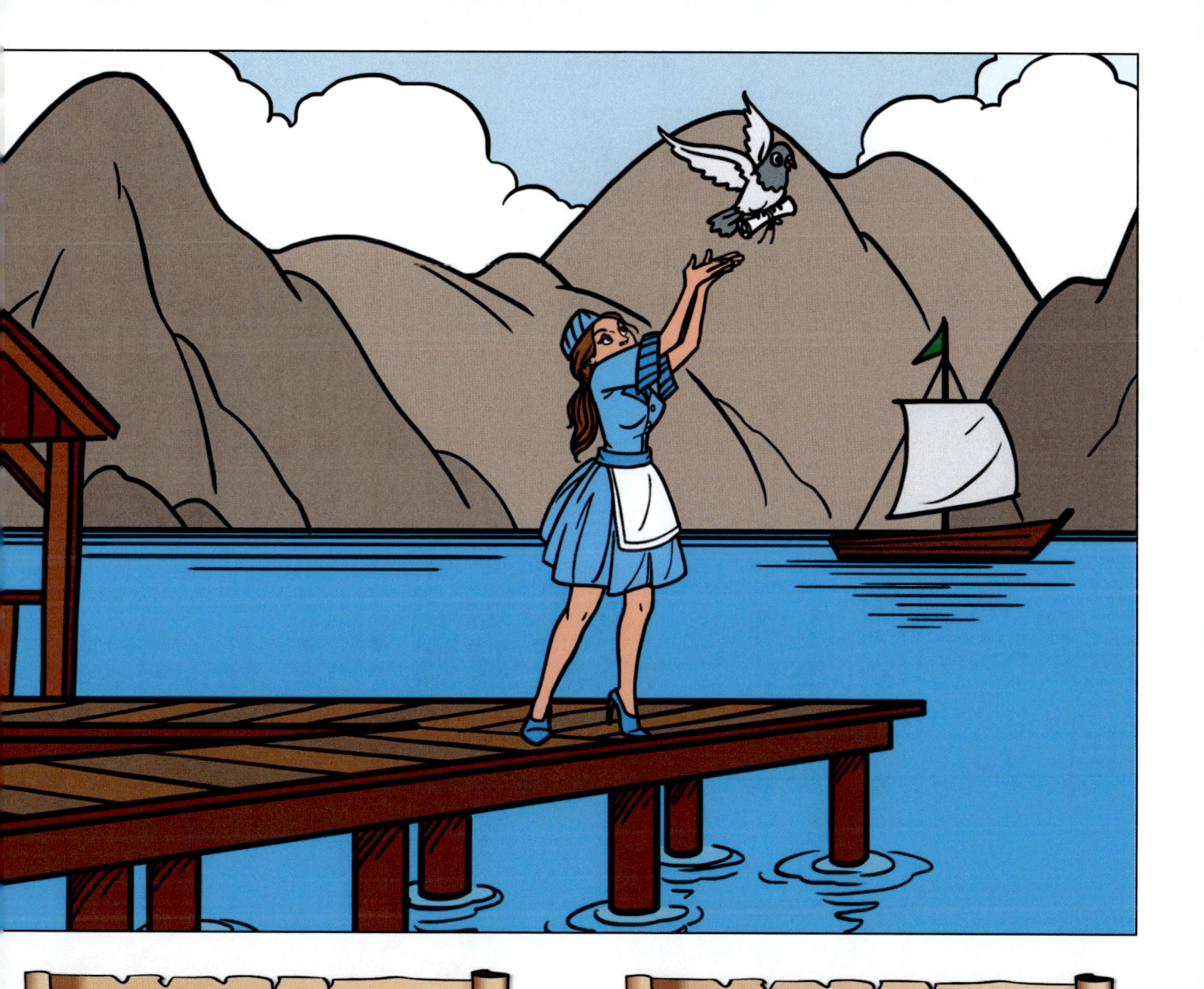

Ŝi subite staris sane,
Ŝajne tute sendolore,
"Vi klopodis min mortigi!"
Diris Katarin' fervore.

"Via kelnerino Minjo
Sendis birdon kun letero.
Ĝi klarigis, ke ŝi donis
Al mi trinkon sen maltero."

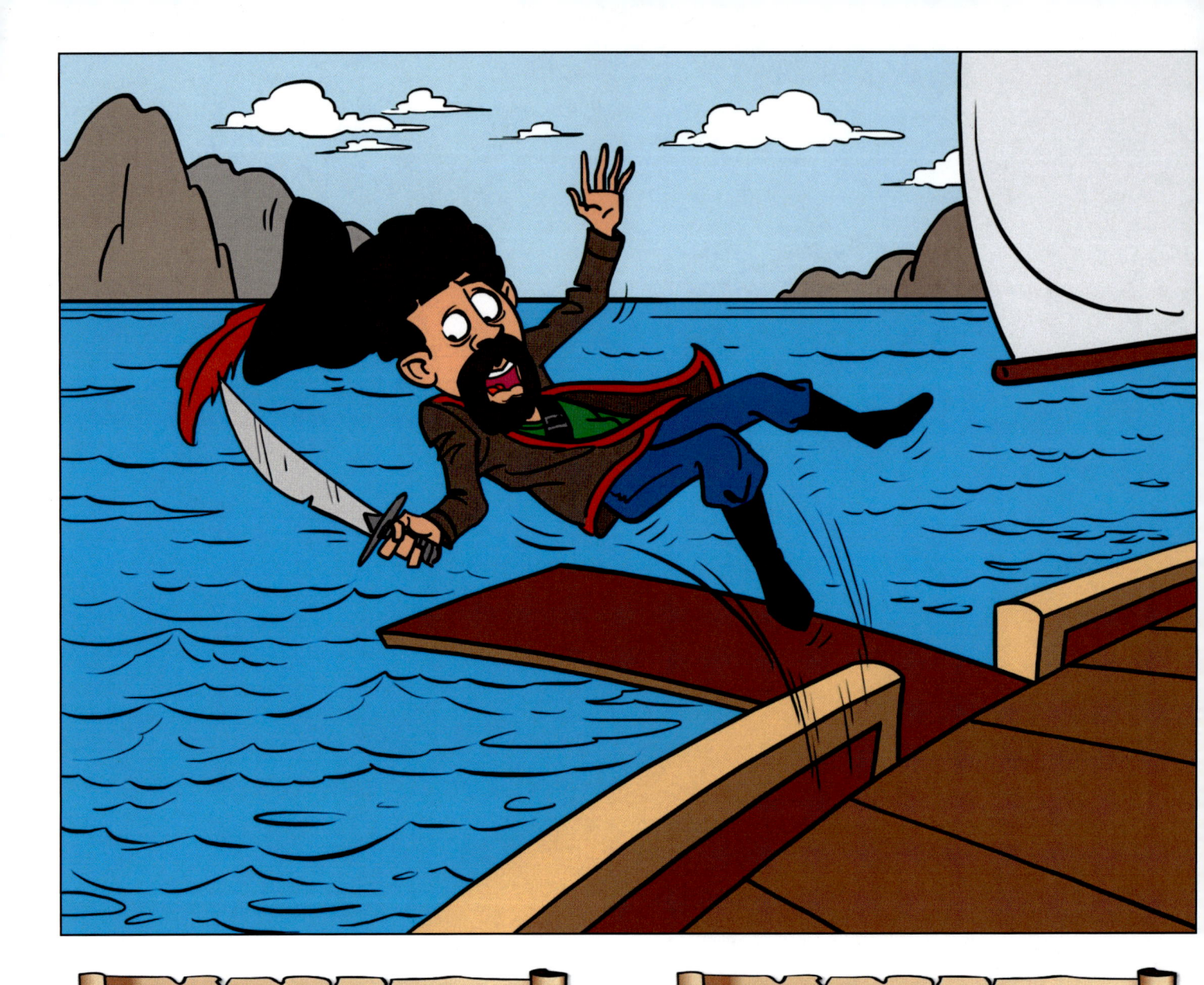

Ŝi malkovris la komploton!
Tuj fariĝis Berto tima!
Li eltiris sian glavon
Kun minaco aĉe krima!

Kun paŝet' li ŝin atakis.
Nun per glav' anstataŭ malte.
Dru' ŝin helpis en la skermo,
Al la paŝtabulo salte.

X

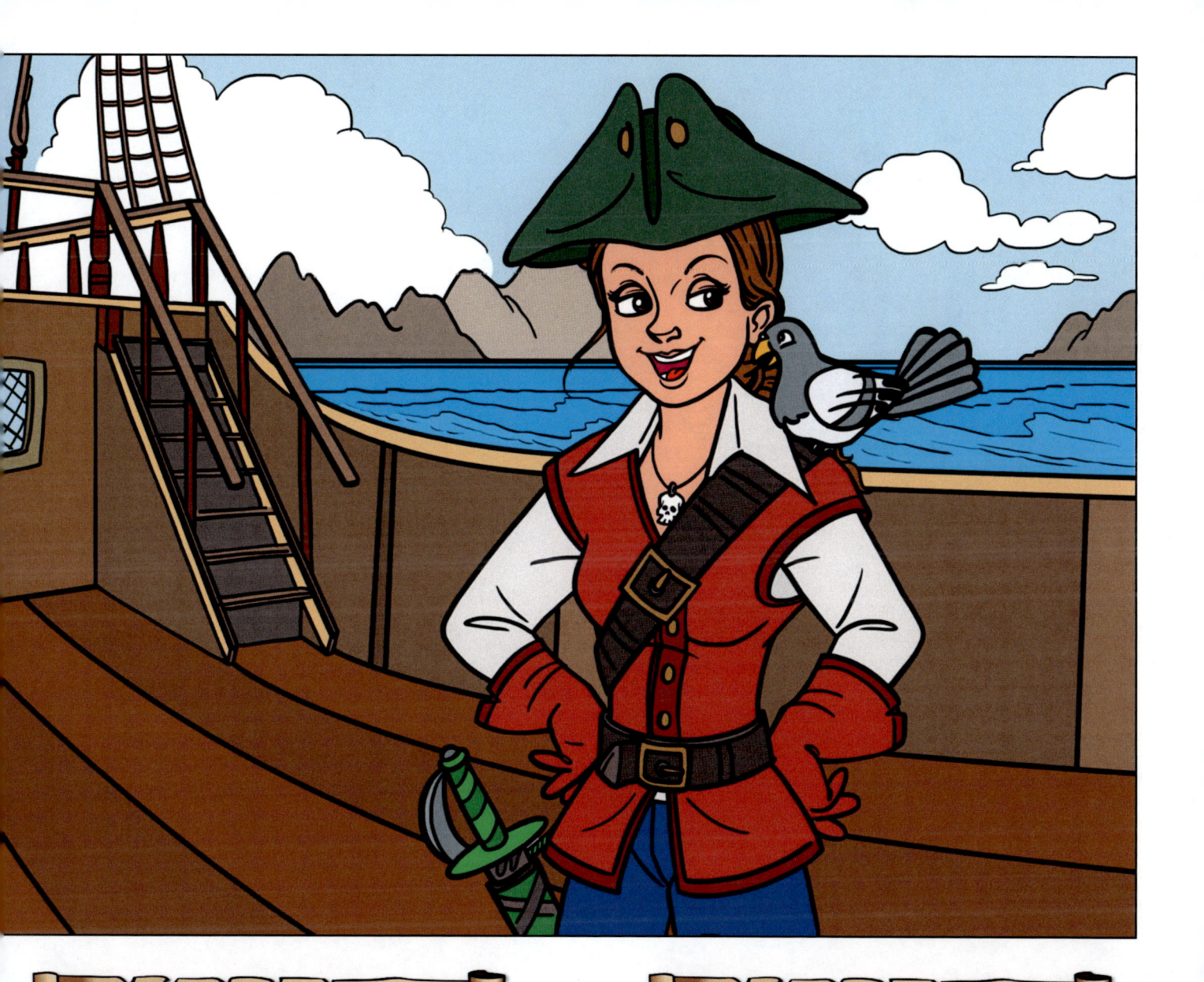

Berto kriis kolerege,
"Venkos mi la kapitanon!"
Li, perdante ekvilibron,
Falis en la oceanon.

Ni neniam trovis Berton,
Ja droninta Berto ŝajnis.
Venontjare estis Minjo,
Kiu la konkurson gajnis.

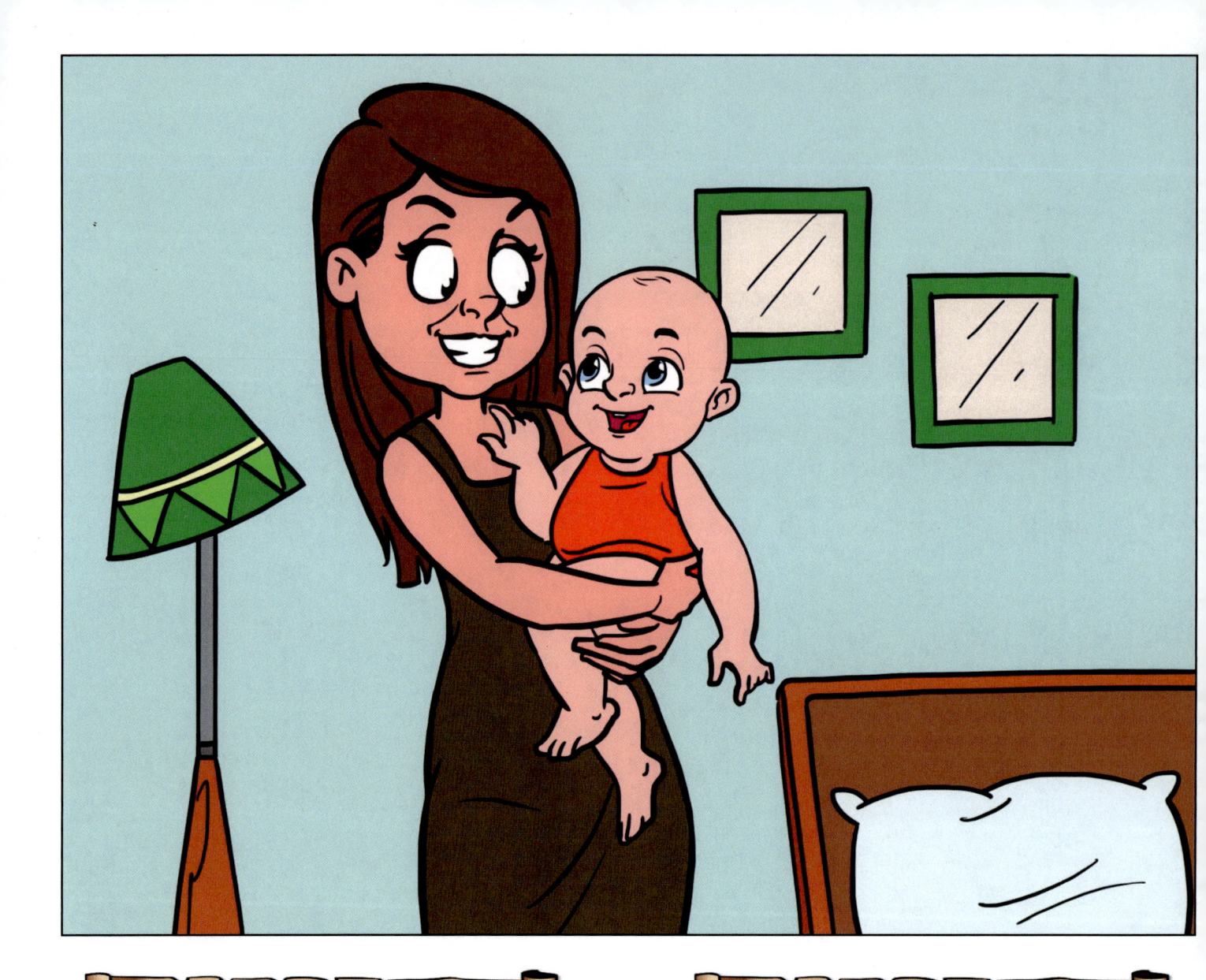

Ne forgesu resti zorga
Pri desertoj kun gluteno.
Ĝi por kelke da amikoj
Estas kiel la veneno.

Baldaŭ beb' troviĝis tie.
Ĝi naskiĝis al Katanjo.
Ŝi sukcesis ja pirate,
Sed elstaris kiel panjo.

A Pirate's Guide to Esperanto!
(All that you need to read this book)

Part One: Letters and Sounds

In Esperanto, every letter always sounds the same (whereas in English a C can sound like an S or a K).
   The letters are never silent so you will hear the K in knabo (whereas in English, the word knight sounds like nite).
Say each vowel separately (so heroo sounds like heh-ROH-oh).

Most of the letters sound just like they do in English. Some of them work a little differently:

C is always like the TS in its
G is always like the hard G in go
J is always like the Y in yes
R is always lightly rolled like it is in Spanish*
S is always like the S in sale (never like the Z sound in as)

Esperanto doesn't use the letters Q, W, X, or Y, but it does have some special ones:

Ĉ is like the CH in chat
Ĝ is like the soft G in giant
Ĥ is like the Scottish CH in loch
Ĵ is like the soft J sound in Asia
Ŝ is like the SH in shut
Ŭ is like the W in win

All the letters:
A B C Ĉ D E F
G Ĝ H Ĥ I J Ĵ
K L M N O P R
S Ŝ T U Ŭ V Z

Vowels are easy to use in Esperanto because they always sound the same no matter where you see them.

This phrase will help you remember the right sounds: "Pa let me go too."

A is like the A in Pa
E is like the E in let
I is like the E in me
O is like the O in go
U is like the OO in too

Here are the vowel combos:

Aŭ is like the OW in cow
Aj is like the IE in lie
Ej is like the AY in day
Oj is like the OY in boy
Uj is like the OOEY in gooey

The Esperanto alphabet is super easy to say!

Instead of ess, are, and tee for S, R, and T, you just stick an O sound after every consonant so they all sound alike. S, R, and T sound like so, row, and toe.

   I hope you enjoy the letter N (in English: en), but there's no sound like the letter N (in Esperanto: no).

   Each vowel's name is simply their vowel sound, without any extra sounds before or after them. That means the name for A is like opening your mouth and saying ahh for the doctor during a checkup.

Always emphasize or stress the second-to-last syllable of a word.

Konis is like KOH-neese
Piratoj is like pee-RAH-toy
Katarino is like kah-tah-REE-noh

*If you have trouble rolling your R's, just touch your tongue to the roof of your mouth while making an R and it should sound close enough.

In Esperanto, you can often tell by a word's ending how it is being used in a sentence.

Nouns end in -o   (pirato = a pirate)
Plural nouns end in -oj (piratoj = pirates)
Adjectives end in -a   (bela = beautiful)
Adverbs end in -e   (subite = suddenly)
Infinitives end in -i   (kredi = to believe)
Commands end in -u   (parolu! = speak!)
Conditionals end in -us (estus = would be)

When a noun is the direct object of a sentence and receives the action, it ends with the letter -n.

Virino rabas ŝipo<u>n</u>. = A woman robs a ship.
   (The ship is being robbed so we put ŝipo<u>n</u>.)
Virino<u>n</u> rabas ŝipo. = A ship is robbing a woman.
   (The -n in virino<u>n</u> makes HER the one getting robbed.)

You can often rearrange words without changing a sentence's meaning; -n endings make that possible.
<u>Mi amas vin</u>. <u>Vin amas mi</u>. <u>Vin mi amas</u>. <u>Mi vin amas</u>.
Those four sentences ALL mean "I love you."

In Esperanto, you can build words by adding affixes (beginnings and endings) to them.

<u>Orda</u> means <u>in order</u> and <u>igi</u> means <u>to make it that way</u>.
<u>Ordigi</u> means <u>to clean or organize</u> and <u>-ilo</u> means <u>a tool</u>.
<u>Ordigilo</u> means <u>a cleaning or organizing tool or device</u>.
<u>For</u> means <u>away</u> and <u>ĵeti</u> means <u>to throw</u>.
<u>Forĵeti</u> means <u>to throw away</u>.

An adjective's ending must match the noun it describes, so if the noun ends in -j, -n, or -jn, so does its adjective.

La grand<u>a</u> pirat<u>o</u> ŝatas ŝipojn.   = The big pirate likes ships.
La pirato ŝatas grand<u>ajn</u> ŝip<u>ojn</u>. = The pirate likes big ships.
(See how grand<u>a</u> becomes grand<u>ajn</u> when describing ŝip<u>ojn</u>?)

Part Two: Nouns & Pronouns

Here are what pronouns look like:

Mi = I		mia = my
Vi = you		via = your
Ni = we		nia = our
Li = he		lia = his
Ŝi = she		ŝia = her
Ĝi = it		ĝia = its
Ili = they (a specific group)		ilia = their
Oni = they (as in "you know what they say")			

The direct object form is made by adding -n to a pronoun.

Min = me
Vin = you   Mi amas ŝin.
Nin = us   I love her.
Lin = him
Ŝin = her   Ŝi amas lin.
Ĝin = it   She loves him.
Ilin = them

Esperanto has no indefinite article (a, an).
Urbo = a city   La urbo = the city
Fino = an end   La fino = the end

The special pronoun <u>si</u> means oneself or one's own instead of somebody else's.
<u>Li ŝatas lin.</u> = <u>He likes him (another man).</u>
<u>Li ŝatas sin.</u> = <u>He likes himself.</u>
<u>Li vendis lian ŝipon.</u> = <u>He sold that guy's ship.</u>
<u>Li vendis sian ŝipon.</u> = <u>He sold his own ship.</u>

When a noun has two -o words like *Kapitano Katarino*, only the first -o word ever gets that special -n ending.

Kapitano Katarino amas mi<u>n</u>.   = Captain Katie loves me.
Kapitano<u>n</u> Katarino amas mi.   = I love Captain Katie.
Tio kolerigis Kapitano<u>n</u> Katarino. = That angered Captain Katie.

All verbs in Esperanto work the same way!
Learn how to use one verb, and you can use them all!

> **Part Three: Verbs**

Esperanto verbs can end in -is, -as, or -os which means past, present, or future.
Remember the name P<u>icasso</u> to keep the past, present, and future vowels in order.

Li vend<u>is</u> = He <u>sold</u>	Ŝi leg<u>is</u> = She <u>read</u>	Ili lud<u>is</u> = They <u>played</u>
Li vend<u>as</u> = He <u>sells</u>	Ŝi leg<u>as</u> = She <u>reads</u>	Ili lud<u>as</u> = They <u>play</u>
Li vend<u>os</u> = He <u>will sell</u>	Ŝi leg<u>os</u> = She <u>will read</u>	Ili lud<u>os</u> = They <u>will play</u>

Verbs can be turned into *participles* which are words that describe what a person or thing <u>was</u>/<u>is</u>/<u>will be</u> doing or what <u>has been</u>/<u>is being</u>/<u>will be</u> done to them.

The endings <u>-into</u>, <u>-anto</u>, and <u>-onto</u> mean one who <u>was</u>, <u>is</u>, or <u>will be</u> actively doing something.
A person who was reading? Leg<u>into</u>.   Is reading? Leg<u>anto</u>.   Will be reading? Leg<u>onto</u>.

The endings <u>-ito</u>, <u>-ato</u>, and <u>-oto</u> mean one who <u>was</u>, <u>is</u>, or <u>will be</u> passively receiving an action.
A person who got captured? Kapt<u>ito</u>.   Is getting captured? Kapt<u>ato</u>.   Will get captured? Kapt<u>oto</u>.

You can use an -a ending to turn these words into descriptive adjectives.
<u>Renkontita viro</u>   = <u>A met man.</u>   (A man that someone has met or come across)
<u>Li estas leganta libron.</u> = <u>He is reading a book.</u> (Or you could just say "Li legas libron" instead)
<u>Mi havas legotan libron.</u> = <u>I have a will-be-read book.</u>

When you stack verbs together,
all but one of them should end in -i.

Venu!	= Come!
Bonvolu veni!	= Please come!
Bonvolu provi veni!	= Please try to come!
Mi hezitas provi manĝi.	= I hesitate to try to eat.
Mi devis voli dormi.	= I had to want to sleep.

It's different when there's a *ke* between them.
Mi petas, ke vi manĝu.   = I request that you eat.

Devus might be the trickiest verb in Esperanto.
It looks like it means "would have the duty to"
but it simply means "should" or "ought to."

Mi devis manĝi.	= I had to eat.
Mi devas manĝi.	= I have to eat.
Mi devos manĝi.	= I will have to eat.
Mi devus manĝi.	= I should eat.

Any other time you see the -us ending, it means "would _____," so 'Mi legus' means "I would read."

Sometimes a sentence will sound weird in English if you translate everything word-for-word, but it makes perfect sense in Esperanto all together.

"<u>Mi devus manĝi</u>"   means "I should eat,"   not "<u>I ought to to eat</u>"
"<u>Mi ne ĝin povas manĝi</u>" means "I can't eat it,"   not "<u>I not it is able to to eat</u>"
"<u>Devas vi eviti ion</u>"   means "You have to avoid something," not "<u>Must you to avoid something</u>"

> # Part Four:
> # Final Tips and Trivia

A final -o ending can often be taken out and replaced with an apostrophe.

This means that vir<u>o</u> can become vir' but vir<u>on</u> and vir<u>oj</u> cannot be shortened.

<u>Atak'</u> = <u>Atako</u> (These both mean <u>an attack</u>)
<u>La firmeco de la vir'</u> = <u>La firmeco de la viro</u>

This doesn't change where the stress goes in the word.
<u>Kajako</u> and <u>kajak'</u> = <u>kie-YAHK-oh</u> and <u>kie-YAHK</u>

<u>La</u> can be shortened to <u>l'</u> when it comes after a preposition like <u>de</u> which ends in a vowel:
ĉe l' = ĉe la   de l' = de la   je l' = je la

La nupto de l' viro = La nupto de la viro
(They both mean <u>the marriage of the man</u>.)

The -n ending can indicate a frequency or period of time as well as a direct object.

Mi manĝas ĉiun tagon.	= I eat every day.
Mi manĝas pomon.	= I eat an apple.
Ĉiun tagon mi manĝas pomon.	= Every day I eat an apple.

Sometimes the -n ending means motion toward.

Ŝi ĵetis ĝin planken.	= She threw it toward the floor.
Li falis suben.	= He fell down below.
Saltu sur la tablo.	= Jump on the table.
Saltu sur la tablo<u>n</u>.	= Jump on<u>to</u> the table.
Li iris al sia hejmo.	= He went to his home.
Mi iris hejmen.	= I went home.

The word *Esperanto* means "one who hopes." When Ludwik Zamenhof created the language, he used the pen name *Dr. Esperanto* on his books because when he first tried publishing a new language using his real name years earlier, his father destroyed all his work!

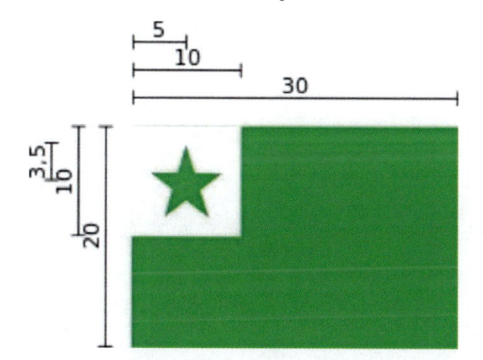

This is the flag of Esperanto. The numbers show exactly how big the star and canton (white part) should be and where they belong.
Green is the official color of Esperanto.

Some Esperanto Affixes

bo- (in-law)	bopatro (father-in-law)
ek- (sudden or momentary)	ekvidi (to suddenly see)
ge- (includes both genders)	geedzoj (spouses)
mal- (opposite)	malgranda (small)
re- (again)	revenis (came back again)
-adi (continuous action)	ludadi (to keep playing)
-aĵo (substance or thing)	bakaĵo (a baked good)
-ano (a member)	urbano (citizen)
-ĉjo (male nickname)	Patro -> Paĉjo (Daddy)
-eco (quality of something)	firmeco (firmness)
-ego (intensifies, very...)	miltego (a huge war)
-ejo (a place for something)	bakejo (a bakery)
-eto (minimizes, a little...)	ŝipeto (a little ship)
-igi (to cause or make...)	feliĉigi (to make happy)
-iĝi (to become...)	feliĉiĝi (to become happy)
-ilo (a tool or instrument)	sonorilo (a bell)
-ino (feminine version)	reĝino (a queen)
-inda (worthy of...)	leginda (worth reading)
-isto (a professional)	bakisto (a baker)
-njo (female nickname)	Patrino -> Panjo (Mommy)
-ujo (a container)	panujo (a breadbox)
-ulo (a person who is...)	junulo (a young person)

* Here are all the Esperanto words used in this book *

Aĉe (horribly, wretchedly)
Aĵo (a physical material or substance)
Al (to or toward)
Amiko (a friend)
Anstataŭ (instead of)
Atakis (attacked)
Aŭdis (heard)
Aŭskulti (to listen) / **Aŭskultu** (Listen!)
Baldaŭ (soon)
Bebo (a baby)
Berto or **Bert'** (Robert, the bad guy in the story)
Birdo (a bird)
Bronzo (bronze which here means a third-place trophy)
Certe (certainly, surely, definitely)
Ĉiam (always)
Ĉesos (will cease, will stop, will end)
Ĉu (Creates "yes or no" questions or means "whether")
  Ĉu mi kuris? = Did I run?   Ĉu vere? = Really?
  Li scias, ĉu mi kuris. = He knows whether I ran.
Eĉ (even as in "I can't even")
Ekvilibro (balance, equilibrium)
Eltiris (drew out; el-tiri "to pull out")
Danki (to thank) / **Dankon** (Thanks!)
De (of or from)
Decidis (decided)
Demandis (asked or questioned)
Deserto (a dessert, a treat)
Detrui (to destroy or ruin)
Devas (must or "has to")
Devus (should or "ought to")
Diris (said or told)
Do (so or therefore)
Donis (did give) / **Donus** (would give)
Doloro (a pain)
Doloregus (dolor-eg-us "would greatly hurt")
Drinkado (drink-ado "continuous alcohol drinking")
Droninta (drowned, dead from staying under water)
Druo or **Dru'** (Andrew or Drew, the husband of Katie)
Du (two) / **Dum** (during or while)
Durumo (durum, a type of wheat with gluten in it)
Eble (possibly, perhaps)
Edzo (a husband)
Eksteren (toward outside)
Elstaris (excelled, stood out; el-stari "to stand out")
Eltrovus (would find out; el-trovi "to find out")
En (in or into)

Enhavas (includes; en-havas "has inside it...")
Estas (is or "it is...") / **Estis** (was or "it was...")
Fakto (a fact)
Falis (fell)
Fariĝis (became; far-iĝi "to become...")
Faruna (flour-related, having to do with flour)
Fervore (fervently, strongly, passionately)
Fino or **Fin'** (a finish, a finale, or an end)
Forgesi (to forget)
Forgesu (forget!)
Fortrinkis (drank up; for-trinki "to drink it all away")
Gajno (a gain, win, or victory) / **Gajnis** (won)
Glaciaĵo (ice cream; glaci-aĵo "an icy thing")
Glasopleno (glaso-pleno "a glass-full")
Glavo (a sword)
Gluteno (gluten)
Graveda (pregnant, going to have a baby)
Ĝoji (to be joyful) / **Ĝojis** (was overjoyed)
Havus (were to have, theoretically had)
Helpis (helped)
Hontis (was ashamed)
Hordeo (barley, a type of grain with gluten in it)
Hospitalo (a hospital, a place for sick people)
Interese (interestingly, or, by itself, "That's interesting")
Informi (to inform)
Iri (to go) / **Iris** (went)
Ja (indeed)
Je (a special word that can mean *at*, *to*, *regarding*, etc.)
Jen (means "Behold!" or "Here is..." or "It is...")
Kaj (and)
Kapitano (a captain)
Katarino (Katherine)
Katanjo (Katie; the nickname form of Katherine)
Ke (that as in "I know that you are")
Kelke da (a few of, some, several)
Kelnerino (a waitress; kelner-in-o "a female waiter")
Kiel (how or like) / **Kiel ajn** (however at all)
Kien (whither or "to where")
Kirlaĵo (a milkshake; kirl-aĵ-o "a swirled substance")
Kiu (who or which)
Klarigis (clarified; klar-igi "to make clear")
Klopodis (tried, endeavored, took steps to...)
Kolerege (angrily, wrathfully)
Kolerigis (enraged; koler-igi "to make angry")
Kompatinda (poor, pitiful, worthy of compassion)
Komploto (a plot, a conspiracy)
Komprenus (would understand)
Konas (knows or "is familiar with")

Konkurso (a competition such as a race)
Konkursado (regular or continual competing)
Kontraŭ (against)
Koro (a heart)
Kriis (exclaimed, cried out)
Krima (criminal, illegal)
Kuiristo (a cook; kuir-isto "a professional cooker")
Kun (with)
Kunmiksi (to blend; kun-miksi "to mix together")
La (the)
Lakto (milk)
Letero (a letter as in "a letter in the mail")
Malgajno (a loss; mal-gajno "the opposite of a win")
Malkovrinte (having discovered…)
Malkovris (discovered; mal-kovri "opposite of to cover")
Malto (malt, a form of grain which goes in or on candy)
Malta (malted or related to malt)
Maltaĵo (a malted milkshake; malt-aĵo "a malt thing")
Malte (by using malt)
Maltero (malt-ero "a tiny piece or particle of malt")
Manĝo (a meal)
Mano (a hand)
Mendis (ordered like "he ordered a meal")
Minaco (a threat or menace)
Minjo (Mia, the nickname form of Amelia)
Montris (showed, displayed)
Mortigi (to kill; mort-igi "to make dead")
Naskiĝis (was born; nask-iĝi "to be born")
Ne (no or not)
Neniam (never)
Nun (now)
Nur (only)
Oceano (an ocean; "en la oceanon" = "into the ocean")
Oro (gold which here means a first-place trophy)
Panjo (a mom; the nickname form of patrino or mother)
Paŝo (a step) / **Paŝeto** (a little step)
Paŝtabulo (a gangplank for walking on)
Pensi (to think)
Pensis (thought as in "he thought")
Per ("by way of" or "by using")
Perdante (perd-ante "while losing…")
Pirata (pirate-related) / **Pirato** (a pirate)
Pirate (pirately or "as a pirate")
Piratŝipo (pirat-ŝipo "a pirate ship")
Por ("for" or "in order to")
Poste (afterward)
Povas (currently can) / **Povus** (theoretically could)
Premio (a prize or trophy)

Pri (about or "in regards to")
Pro (as a result of, because of)
Resti (to remain or stay)
Ridis (laughed)
Rivalo (a rival, a competitor, an opponent)
Salte (with a leap)
Sano (health) / **Sane** (healthfully or "in good health")
Se (if)
Sed (but)
Sekalo (rye, a type of grain with gluten in it)
Sen (without)
Sendolore (painlessly; sen-dolore "without pain")
Sendis (did send) / **Sendus** (theoretically would send)
Senglutena (gluten-free; sen-glutena "without gluten")
Simple (simply)
Sincere (sincerely, truly, honestly)
Skermo (a skirmish, a sword fight)
Staris (stood)
Subite (suddenly)
Sukcesis (succeeded)
Ŝajne (seemingly) / **Ŝajnis** (seemed, appeared to be)
Ŝipkonkurso (a ship race)
Tago (a day)
Teni (to hold) / **Tenis** (held)
Termino (a term, word, or expression)
Tie (there)
Tima (timid, afraid)
Tio (that as in "I like that")
Tiu (that as in "I like that one" or "I like that person")
Toleri (to tolerate, to be able to handle)
Tosto (a toast, a speech you give before a drink)
Tre (very or very much)
Trinki (to drink something)
Trinkaĵo (a drink like water, tea, or a malted milkshake)
Trinko (a drink like the action of taking a drink)
Tritiko (wheat, which has gluten in it)
Trovi (to find) / **Troviĝas** (trov-iĝas "is found")
Tuj (immediately)
Tute (totally)
Uzas (uses)
Venena (poisonous) / **Veneno** (a poison or venom)
Venko (a victory)
Venkos (will vanquish or defeat)
Venontjare (during the next year…)
Vere (truly)
Viroj (men)
Vundebleco (a weakness or way to be hurt)
Zorga (careful or mindful)

Who Speaks Esperanto?

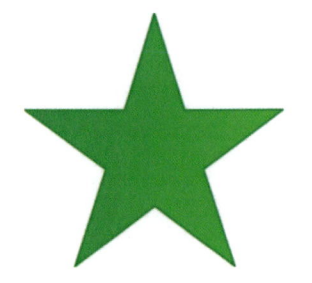

You'll find French speakers in France and German speakers in Germany.

Where can you find other Esperantists??
The answer? In France and Germany AND over 100 other countries!

There are Esperanto clubs in cities all over the world.

Speaking Esperanto gives you thousands of new friends to talk to and visit! Check this out:

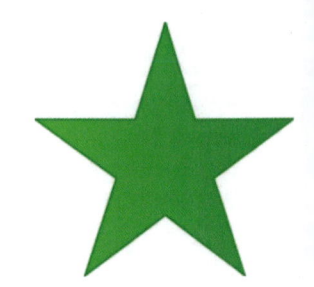

Here's a list of friends who not only speak Esperanto, but donated money to help make this book possible. Dankon!

Rei	Tanja Orme	Matthew Oates
Brandon Sowers	John Cunningham	Annette Brasor
Jorge Rafael Nogueras	Katherine Lister	Zeth Lilliston
João Romero	Marcus	France Gamble
Benson Smith	Ŝono	Mako Allen
Jason Mundy	Rachel Helps	Derek Roff
Paul Lee	Stefan Grotz	James Carroll
Barbara Brown	Nick Platt	Catie Neilson
Erin Legate	Seth Carter	Thomas Warriner

Here are some things to say when you first meet an Esperantist:

Greetings!	= Saluton!	sah-LOO-tone
Welcome!	= Bonvenon!	bone-VEH-known
My name is Lucy.	= Mi nomiĝas Lusi.	mee no-MEE-jahs LOO-see
What did you say?	= Kion vi diris?	KEE-own vee DEE-reese
How are you doing?	= Kiel vi fartas?	KEE-ell vee FAR-tahs
I'm doing well.	= Mi fartas bone.	mee FAR-tahs BOE-neh
Do you want milk?	= Ĉu vi volas lakton?	choo vee VOE-lahs LOCK-tone
Yes! Well, actually, no.	= Jes! Nu, fakte, ne.	yes noo FAHK-teh neh
What a beautiful ostrich!	= Kia bela struto!	KEE-ah BELL-ah STREW-toe
Thanks, friend!	= Dankon, amiko!	DAHN-cone ah-MEE-koe
See you later!	= Ĝis la revido!	JEESE la rev-VEE-doe

Made in United States
Orlando, FL
22 June 2023

34428943R00024